THE MEDICAL CARE OF TERMINALLY ILL PATIENTS

The Johns Hopkins Series in Hematology/Oncology

Jerry L. Spivak, M.D., and Martin D. Abeloff, M.D.,
Consulting Editors

*Supportive Care of Children with Cancer: Current Therapy and Guidelines
from the Children's Cancer Group*
Edited by Arthur R. Ablin, M.D.

Protein Blood Group Antigens of the Human Red Cell
Edited by Peter C. Agre, M.D., and Jean-Pierre Cartron, Ph.D.

*The Hematopoietic Microenvironment: The Functional and Structural Basis of
Blood Cell Development*
Edited by Michael W. Long, Ph.D., and Max S. Wicha, M.D.

Cancer Treatment and the Heart
Edited by Franco Muggia, M.D., Michael D. Green, M.D., and
James L. Speyer, M.D.

The Fundamentals of Clinical Hematology, third edition
Edited by Jerry L. Spivak, M.D., and Edward R. Eichner, M.D.

THE MEDICAL CARE
OF TERMINALLY
ILL PATIENTS

ROBERT E. ENCK, M.D.

Clinical Assistant Professor, Department of Medicine
Ohio State University School of Medicine

Editor-in-Chief
American Journal of Hospice and Palliative Care

The Johns Hopkins University Press / Baltimore and London

© 1994 The Johns Hopkins University Press
All rights reserved
Printed in the United States of America on acid-free paper
03 02 01 00 99 98 97 96 95 94   5 4 3 2

The Johns Hopkins University Press
2715 North Charles Street
Baltimore, Maryland 21218-4319
The Johns Hopkins Press Ltd., London

Readers should scrutinize product information sheets for dosage changes or contraindications, particularly for new or infrequently used drugs.

Illustrations were done by Anne Vega.

Library of Congress Cataloging-in-Publication Data

Enck, Robert E.
    The medical care of terminally ill patients / Robert E. Enck.
        p.   cm. — (The Johns Hopkins series in hematology/oncology)
    Includes bibliographical references and index.
    ISBN 0-8018-4675-7 (hc : alk. paper). — ISBN 0-8018-4763-X (pbk : alk. paper)
    1. Terminal care.   I. Title.   II. Series.
    [DNLM: 1. Terminal Care.   2. Palliative Treatment.   WB 310 E56m
1994]
    R726.8.E53   1994
    362.1′75—dc20
    DNLM/DLC
    for Library of Congress   93-20529

A catalog record for this book is available from the British Library.

How people die remains in the memories of those who live on.
Cicely Saunders, "Pain and Impending Death"

Contents

Preface

Before the 1970s, little research had been done to guide the clinician caring for dying patients. Medical management was often dictated by the clinician's prior experience, and what was published in the medical literature was often anecdotal in nature. Treatment with corticosteroids, with or without adequate control of pain and symptoms, was generally the norm. Clinicians perceived palliative care as indicating a failure on their part to cure the underlying disease. Whatever the specialty, physicians were not trained in this area, and fellowships in palliative care were nonexistent.

The emergence of the hospice movement in the early 1980s clearly focused for the public the medical community's deficiencies in dealing with pain and symptom control in dying patients. The major impetus in the United States for hospice care came from outside the medical community and, to some degree, forced physicians to become knowledgeable and humane in treating dying patients. By the middle to late 1980s, new medical journals published articles specifically on the control of pain and symptoms. More importantly, however, this area became a fertile subject for research, in part because of the increasing incidence of cancer and other chronic diseases in the aging population and in part because of the plateauing of effective, curative therapies for these diseases. A good example of this expanding research is the study of megestrol acetate for the treatment of cancer-related anorexia and cachexia, done in a prospective fashion by a cooperative clinical trial group (the North Central Cancer Treatment Group and the Mayo Clinic) sponsored by the National Cancer Institute. More recently, the issue of euthanasia and the commercial success of *Final Exit* have kept the pressure on the medical community to be knowledgeable and compassionate in treating dying patients.

This book represents the efforts of a clinician writing for other clinicians. It was designed to be practical, and it provides a scientific understanding of and subsequent applicability to the management of the complex clinical problems encountered in dying patients. The book is not an all-encompassing encyclopedia on the subject of terminal care and therefore does not quote copious references. Rather, it cites and reviews only those results that are applicable at the bedside. Anecdotal published information is used only occasionally, with emphasis again on the results of sound clinical research.

Generally, incurable diseases exhibit three distinct periods. In the initial, or stable, period, the patient experiences few symptoms and longevity ranges from years to months, as with dementia or motor neuron disease. The second, or symptomatic, period, is characterized by a worsening of the underlying disease, associated with frequent symptoms and a survival of months to weeks. The final, or twilight, period is the dying phase, during which survival is measured in weeks to days and the control of symptoms is more difficult. This book focuses on these last two time spans, when symptoms are common and often interrelated.

The list of symptoms in this book does not include all of the clinical problems found in dying patients; rather, it reflects those the clinician will encounter most frequently. Without question, pain is the major symptom. For this reason, one-third of the book is devoted to this subject. Symptoms such as nausea and vomiting, anorexia and cachexia, constipation, delirium, depression, dyspnea, urinary incontinence, and pressure sores are grouped together because they occur frequently, regardless of the underlying disease. Likewise, problems specific to cancer, namely, malignant intestinal obstruction, malignant dysphagia, neuromuscular dysfunction, and malignant ulceration, are grouped into a single chapter. Also, incurable diseases other than cancer which cause pain and symptoms, such as dementia, motor neuron disease, acquired immunodeficiency syndrome (AIDS), and others, are discussed separately.

This book is organized to provide the reader with a ready resource to enhance his or her knowledge concerning the management of dying patients. I encourage readers to scan the references cited if they seek more detailed information in a specific area. I hope that hospices and palliative care units will find this book useful, as will physicians and nurses, regardless of their experience and level of training, who are faced with the complexities of caring for dying patients as part of their practices.

Acknowledgments

Writing a book is not an easy task, and this book could not have been completed without the enduring support of my family and friends. Although my wife, Martha, and our three sons, Garrett, Gavin, and Gannon, often tired of hearing about "the book," their encouragement and support were never ending. And yes, Gannon, you'll get the first copy.

My parents, Herbert and Birdine Enck, both died of cancer within a short time of each other. Caring for them helped me clearly understand the exhausting pressure and emotional turmoil inflicted on the caregiver coping with a dying patient. Because they both suffered needlessly with poorly controlled symptoms, I felt compelled to write this book for physicians and nurses so that a ready resource for the management of pain and symptoms would be available and others might die more peacefully. Certainly, the memories of an agonizing death of a loved one linger forever.

Wilbur W. Oaks, M.D., was the chief of medicine (1973–83) during my internship and residency at Hahnemann Medical College and Hospital and continues there as professor of medicine. By his caring manner, he makes every patient feel special, whether he spends five minutes or an hour with that patient. He has received many awards and honors for his unique teaching skills, and those of us fortunate enough to be associated with him are really the ones who are honored. He taught me the humanity of medicine.

I also wish to acknowledge the significant support that the Joint Commission on Accreditation of Healthcare Organizations (JCAHO) has given to palliative care, initially in developing standards and an accreditation program for hospice care (1984–89) and then in folding these concepts into its accreditation programs for hospitals, long-term care, and home care. The insight and leadership for these standards come from James S. Roberts, M.D., senior vice president of the JCAHO. Dr. Roberts's strong belief that dying patients have rights including access to high-quality terminal care has significantly improved the lives of countless patients and their families.

In addition, I thank the numerous researchers who have published scientific articles in the area of palliative care. The general lack of funding for research in this area attests to the dedication of these individuals to improving the care of the dying patient.

Special thanks go to my secretary, Marilyn Ann Valois, who truly understands procrastinators, such as I. Robert and Anne Vega were very helpful in producing the illustrations. The reviewers of the manuscript made useful and informative suggestions for improving the format. Finally, I thank Wendy Harris, of the Johns Hopkins University Press, for her encouragement and patience during the course of this project.

THE MEDICAL CARE OF TERMINALLY ILL PATIENTS

Chapter 1

The Prognostication of Survival

The question of accurate prognosis has plagued hospice programs since the Medicare hospice benefit was enacted in 1982. The legislation provides Medicare coverage for terminally ill patients who are certified by physicians to have a prognosis of six months or less to live. An inaccurate prognosis (i.e., the patient lives more than six months) results in a financial drain on the hospice. Shorter survivals (in the range of days), which are commonly encountered, deprive the patient and family of the true benefits of a hospice program. Indeed, as part of a national survey of nonparticipating hospices, the U.S. General Accounting Office indicated that one of the main concerns that led these hospices to choose not to participate in Medicare was the fact that the language required in hospice certification of terminal illnesses related to the certainty of the physician's prognosis of death (U.S. General Accounting Office 1989). As a practical matter, many patients and families need to have some estimation of survival so the patient can get his or her affairs in order and allow appropriate time for good-byes.

In 1949, Karnofsky and Burchenal derived a numerical scale for quantifying a patient's functional status. This scale, now known as the Karnofsky Performance Status (KPS) scale, ranges from 0 to 100:

100 = normal; no complaints, no evidence of disease
 90 = able to carry on normal activity; minor signs or symptoms of
      disease
 80 = able to carry on normal activity with effort; some signs or symp-
      toms of disease
 70 = cares for self but is unable to carry on normal activity or do
      active work
 60 = requires occasional assistance but is able to care for most of his
      or her needs
 50 = requires considerable assistance and frequent medical care
 40 = disabled; requires special care and assistance

30 = severely disabled; hospitalization is indicated, although death is
        not imminent
20 = very sick; hospitalization (active supportive treatment) is neces-
        sary
10 = moribund; fatal processes, progressing rapidly
 0 = dead

In 1985, Evans and McCarthy reported the results of their prognostic studies in 42 terminally ill patients. The six members of a terminal
care support team in a London health district reported both the upper
and the lower estimates of prognosis, in days, on 42 patients during 149
visits, in addition to assessing the KPS score. The authors found that
patients with KPS scores above 50 had a predicted survival of 24 days
and those with scores of 50 or less survived 3 to 70 days. Just over half of
the actual survivals were within the estimated time, which tended to be
overly optimistic. Evans and McCarthy concluded that KPS scores correlated more closely with actual survivals than did estimates provided
by members of the terminal care support team.

Cancer

In 1980, Yates, Chalmer, and McKegney evaluated patients with
advanced cancer using the KPS measurement. They studied 104 patients (42 women and 62 men, with an average age of 57 years). They
collected a KPS score for each patient and then compared the score to
the survival. It was clear that a low KPS score was strongly correlated
with death within a relatively short time. Only 1 of the patients with a
KPS score less than 50 survived longer than six months. However, a
high KPS score was not predictive of long-term survival because many
of the patients with high initial scores died quickly. In addition, a
patient's deterioration and subsequent death within a few months was
predicted, to a limited degree, by a rapidly dropping KPS score.

In 1988 and 1989 Forster and Lynn reported the results of a study
predicting survival for hospice inpatients. In their first paper (1988),
two oncologists, a general internist, an oncology nurse, and a hospice
social worker independently estimated the life span of 108 consecutive
applicants for inpatient hospice care. The survival estimations were
based on data in a 10-page multidisciplinary application packet. The
actual median survival of the 108 patients was 3.5 ± 12.4 weeks. More
than one-fourth of the patients died within 1 week of applying for
hospice care, and only a small proportion lived beyond 12 weeks. The
mean age of the sample was 66.2 years. Slightly more than half were

women, and approximately the same proportion were white. The most common major symptoms and signs at the time of application were ambulation difficulties, anemia, and pain. The survival predictions of the five member groups exceeded the actual survival by an average of 3.4 weeks. The authors speculated that this imprecision in expert estimation of life span poses substantial problems for hospice programs and policy makers.

In their second paper, Forster and Lynn (1989) extended their prior study. The authors collected data on 48 objective patient variables. They were particularly interested in defining objective variables that could distinguish between patients who were likely to die within either three or six months and those who were likely to live longer. These variables included primary neoplasm, hormone treatment, congestive heart failure, pain, disorientation, lack of funds, KPS score, respiratory disease, sodium, admission to hospice, no admission to hospice, weakness, and sex. The KPS score and indication of weakness were the only two variables by logistic regression that contributed substantially to the probability of dying within three months. Using the six-month survival, the investigators found a correlation between women and those who had hormone treatments, indicating a high probability of living beyond six months.

Forster and Lynn (1989) suggested, based upon this survival analysis and their research, that definable groups of applicants to hospice experienced different patterns of survival. They found a worse life expectancy among those with primary neoplasms involving the lung and colon, with disorientation, without congestive heart failure or hormone treatment, and with low sodium levels. Furthermore, the authors found that accurate prognostication of survival takes more precise knowledge than had been previously appreciated and that accuracy may be too limited for reliable forecasts in individual patients.

In 1988, Reuben, Mor, and Hiris published their research, as part of the National Hospice Study, on clinical symptoms and the length of survival in patients with terminal cancer. The authors examined the correlation of 14 clinical symptoms with survival. The symptoms examined were nausea, dry mouth, anorexia, weight loss, difficulty swallowing, constipation, dizziness, fever, shortness of breath, diarrhea, hemorrhaging, bone pain, severe pain, and moderate or severe disorientation. Performance status was measured using the KPS scale. The sample frame was obtained from the National Hospice Study data set. Fifty-three percent of the study patients were women. The average age was 67 years. The KPS score was assessed by trained interviewers on the basis of their observation of the patients.

The authors reported that performance status was the most important clinical factor in estimating the survival time. Of the 14 clinical symptoms assessed, 5 had independent prognostic value: dyspnea, anorexia, dry mouth, trouble swallowing, and weight loss. Based on these variables, the investigators developed four parametric accelerated time survival models to estimate the survival of patients with combinations of these symptoms and then validated the model on the entire data set. This model was not affected by a patient's age, sex, primary tumor site, or type. Reuben, Mor, and Hiris (1988) noted that their prediction rule seemed to be most valuable in estimating the length of survival for patients in the midlevel (KPS 30–40) and high level (KPS ≥ 50) categories of performance status. In their study, 67 percent of the patients were at midlevel KPS. The predicted median survival time ranged from 36 days for patients with all five symptoms to 115 days for patients with none of the symptoms. Similarly, the predicted median survival time for the 17.5 percent of the patients in the highest KPS category was 54 days if all five symptoms were present and 172 days if none was present. For patients in the lowest KPS category (10–20), survival was poor regardless of the number of symptoms present: the predicted median survival time was 16 days if all five symptoms were present and 53 days if none was present. Hence, Reuben et al. concluded that the value of the model may be less for severely dysfunctional terminally ill patients.

Higginson, Wade, and McCarthy (1990) emphasized the importance of the Karnofsky index as a predictor of survival in terminal care. In their 487 patients, there was a clear trend of shorter survival with reducing mobility. When KPS ratings fell to 50 or below, 93 percent died within three months and 99 percent died within six months (table 1.1).

Table 1.1   Survival Time by Change in Karnofsky Performance Status (KPS) Scale in Cancer Patients

KPS Score	Number of Patients	Survival (Days) after Reaching Each KPS Score		
		Mean	Median	Range
80	5	48.6	52	20–69
70	43	48.1	39	0–175
60	96	43.3	29.5	0–344
50	167	30.9	17	0–491
40	204	20.3	11	0–379
30	169	14.8	6	0–372
20	127	11.9	6	0–365
10	80	10.8	2	0–365

Source: Higginson, Wade, and McCarthy (1990).

Dementia

The survival of patients with dementia of the Alzheimer type (DAT) is highly variable, often ranging from five to eight years. To study the clinical course of patients with DAT and to identify factors prognostic of survival, Walsh, Welch, and Larson (1990) prospectively evaluated and followed 200 outpatients with DAT at a university hospital. The mean age was 73.9 years at the onset of symptoms and 77.6 years at enrollment in the study. The median survival time from the onset of symptoms was 9.3 years, with a range of 1.8 to 16+ years, whereas the median survival time from enrollment in the study was 5.3 years, with a range of 0.2 to 7.2+ years. The severity of the dementia, as measured by the Mini-Mental State Examination (a 0- to 30-point scale, with 0 being the most cognitive impaired and 30 being the least impaired), correlated strongly with the survival time. The median survival time of patients with scores of 18 or less was three years shorter than that of patients with scores above 18. Factors found not to influence survival were the duration of symptoms, sex, depression, restlessness, co-morbid conditions, vision problems, a reported decrease in appetite, the use of prescription drugs, and selected laboratory abnormalities (anemia, a low serum folate level, and an abnormal serum creatinine level).

A multivariate analysis of the age at onset of symptoms and of historical features showed that the combination of wandering and falling and the presence of behavioral problems at the time of evaluation seemed to affect survival adversely. The authors did not expect this finding, since patients with dementia are known to have a higher risk for falls and fractures than nondemented patients of the same age. These fractures often immobilize patients, which in turn leads to other potentially fatal complications, such as pulmonary embolus and aspiration pneumonia. The multivariate analysis suggested that behavioral problems were related to wandering and falling but were not as important in predicting survival. As noted by the authors, behavioral problems themselves and the management of them may be responsible for poor outcomes. For example, the use of sedative and hypnotic drugs to control agitation has been associated with falling and hip fractures (Ray et al. 1987).

Motor Neuron Disease

O'Brien, Kelly, and Saunders (1992) retrospectively evaluated their experience with 124 patients with motor neuron disease cared for at St.

Table 1.2   Survival Time Related to Patient's Age
at the Onset of Motor Neuron Disease

Age at Onset (yr)	Number of Patients	Mean Survival (mo)
<40	3	77
40–49	15	77
50–59	30	48
60–69	43	35
70–79	27	28
≥80	3	13
Total	121[a]	42

Source: O'Brien, Kelly, and Saunders (1992).
[a]Date of death unknown for three patients.

Christopher's Hospice during a 12-year period. The age at the onset of
the illness correlated significantly with survival, with younger patients
living longer than older patients (table 1.2).

Acquired Immunodeficiency Syndrome (AIDS)

Because of the fairly recent onset of the AIDS epidemic, few studies
have systematically evaluated factors prognostic of the length of survival of the terminally ill patient with AIDS. To this end, Cole (1991)
reviewed the medical literature to identify clinically significant indicators for survival (table 1.3). Clearly, there is wide variation in survival
with complicating diseases such as Kaposi sarcoma and non-Hodgkin
lymphoma, which reflects the degree of underlying impairment of the
patient's immune system. For example, the prognosis for Kaposi sarcoma occurring in patients with no concurrent opportunistic infections and little immune dysfunction is more favorable (median survival
of 31 months) than that of the same tumor seen in patients with advanced AIDS (median survival of 7 months).

Central Nervous System Anoxia

Global central nervous system anoxia, often following cardiopulmonary arrest, may lead to a chronic vegetative state, with hopelessness for the family and an array of distressing symptoms for the patient. Longstreth et al. (1983) retrospectively studied the neurologic
sequelae of out-of-hospital cardiac arrest, using 459 consecutive patients admitted to a teaching hospital over ten years. One hundred

Table 1.3   The Prognostic Indicators of Survival Time
in Patients with AIDS

Coexisting Condition	Survival (mo)
Opportunistic infection	
Pneumocystis carinii pneumonia	24 (mean)
Mycobacterium avium intracellulare	7 (median)
Tumor	
Kaposi sarcoma	7–31 (medians)
Non-Hodgkin lymphoma	6.8–24 (medians)
Other complication	
AIDS-related dementia	1.8 (median)
Neurologic abnormalities	2.1 (median)
Constant diarrhea	3.2 (median)
Hypoxia ($pO_2 \leq 50$ mm Hg)	1.0 (median)
Low serum albumin (<20 grams/L)	0.7 (median)
Peripheral blood pancytopenia[a]	2.5 (median)

Source: Cole (1991).

[a]Lymphocytes <1.5 × 10/L, hematocrit <30%, white blood cells <2.5 × 10 9/L, and platelets <140 × 10 9/L.

eighty patients (39 percent) never awakened and 279 (61 percent) awakened, 188 without and 91 with persistent neurologic deficits. Patients who never awoke had a median survival of 3.5 days. The longer a comatose patient survived, the smaller the chance of ever awakening or awakening without deficits. In another study, Levy et al. (1985) investigated the outcome of coma after cardiac arrest in 210 patients and were able to develop simple prognostication rules for this clinical situation. Patients who, with initial examination or after 24 hours, had pupillary light reflexes, the development of spontaneous eye movements, and withdrawal response to pain experienced favorable outcomes.

Advanced Pulmonary Disease

Some 70 to 80 percent of patients with advanced pulmonary disease die within five years (Bergner et al. 1988). As noted by Kinzel (1991), prognostication is even more difficult in patients with advanced lung disease than in patients with cancer. Indeed, one study showed estimates varying from one month to five years in similar patients.

Summary

No matter what the disease, the prognostication of survival is an inexact science widely influenced by individual patient variation. Generally, survival estimates made by physicians and nurses tend to be overly optimistic.

In patients with advanced cancer, a low KPS score usually reflects a life span of a few weeks to days. In the more ambulatory and mobile patients (i.e., those with a middle to high KPS score), accurate prognostication of survival is more difficult. Therefore, like pain assessment, ongoing measurement of KPS scores is an important clinical tool to monitor prognosis, especially as the scores decline.

The survival of patients with dementia of the Alzheimer type is highly variable. The severity of the dementia correlates strongly with survival: patients with milder dementia live significantly longer than do those more severely affected. Also, the presence of behavioral problems and the combination of wandering and falling at the time of the initial evaluation adversely influence survival.

In patients with motor neuron disease, the length of life correlates inversely with the age of onset, with younger patients living longer than older patients.

Survival in patients with AIDS is also variable but seems to relate to the degree of impairment of the immune system. Patients with marked immune dysfunction as evidenced by the presence of opportunistic infections and malignant neoplasms survive for months.

Recovery from central nervous system anoxia after cardiopulmonary arrest directly relates to the patient's initial or 24-hour neurologic status. Improvement in this status denotes a favorable outcome, whereas persisting coma suggests a short survival.

Finally, the prognostication of survival in patients with advanced pulmonary disease is extremely difficult, and survival may range from months to years.

PART I

The Management of Symptoms
Common among Dying Patients

Chapter 2

General Symptoms of Dying Patients

Of all the symptoms encountered in dying patients, pain is the most common. It is discussed extensively in Part II.

GASTROINTESTINAL SYMPTOMS

Nausea and Vomiting

Patients with advanced diseases frequently experience nausea and vomiting. If unabated, these symptoms lead to serious nutritional problems, dehydration, and overall physical discomfort. In patients with cancer, these symptoms are generally associated with the use of chemotherapy. Much research effort has been expended on developing various regimens of antiemetic drugs to control this distressing but time-limited side effect.

What has not been well studied or even well appreciated is the incidence of non-chemotherapy-induced nausea and vomiting in patients dying from advanced cancer. Reuben and Mor (1986b) shed some light on this subject as part of the National Hospice Study, which prospectively followed cancer patients over their last weeks of life. The authors found that 62 percent of patients with terminal cancer experienced nausea and vomiting at some point in the last two months of life. Nausea and vomiting were reported more often in the following groups: patients with stomach or breast cancer as the primary type, women (even after excluding those with breast cancer), and patients younger than 65 years. Approximately 25 percent of the patients in this study were receiving chemotherapy, and no association was observed between the chemotherapy and the reporting of nausea and vomiting at any time during the last six weeks of life. This finding suggests that the pathogenesis of chemotherapy-induced nausea and vomiting may differ from that due to terminal cancer itself. Of the subset of nauseated patients, only 32 percent received an antiemetic prescription for a phenothiazine or an antihistamine. Physicians were more hesitant to prescribe antiemetic drugs for elderly patients and those with impaired levels of awareness. The results of this study imply that better physician awareness may promote earlier therapeutic intervention to help alleviate these symptoms in patients with terminal cancer.

CAUSES

With the recognition and early identification of this problem, attention can be directed toward identifying the various causes of the symptoms and then treating the symptoms. Frequently, the cause of nausea and vomiting in the cancer patient is multifactorial (table 2.1).

Frytak and Moertel (1981) stressed the diagnostic subtleties of several of these causative factors, such as fluid and electrolyte disturbances, hypercalcemia, adrenocortical insufficiency, and meningeal metastases. This etiologic morass is often compounded by the addition of both opioid and nonopioid analgesic drugs to control pain. Indeed, in the World Health Organization's two-year experience with the analgesic ladder in cancer pain, nausea and vomiting were present in 22 percent of the days during the three-step treatment (Ventafridda et al. 1987). Furthermore, it seems that the incidence of nausea and vomiting is markedly increased in ambulatory patients treated with opioid analgesics.

A possible cause for nausea and vomiting may be the presence of the syndrome of cardiovascular autonomic insufficiency (CAI). The clinical spectrum of CAI includes cardiovascular manifestations (postural hypotension, syncope, fixed heart rate) and gastrointestinal symptoms (nausea, anorexia, constipation, diarrhea). This syndrome is usually found in neurologic disorders, chronic renal disease, and diabetes mellitus. However, Bruerea, Chadwick, Fox, et al. (1986) studied a group of breast cancer patients for the presence of CAI and identified this as a frequent feature in advanced cancer. The nausea, mostly chronic in CAI, was attributed to gastroparesis or a significantly prolonged gastric emptying time.

MANAGEMENT

Ideally, the management of nausea and vomiting is dependent on identifying and correcting the underlying causes (e.g., the use of corticosteroids for adrenocortical insufficiency, antibiotics for infections, and the like). In reality, the major problem is that in many cases the causes are multifactorial and often uncorrectable, as in the case of a

Table 2.1   Common Causes of Nausea and Vomiting
in Patients with Advanced Disease

Fluid and electrolyte disturbances
   Hypercalcemia
   Volume depletion
   Water intoxication (syndrome of inappropriate ADH[a] secretion)
   Adrenocortical insufficiency
Gastrointestinal causes
   Mouth: infections (*Candida albicans*, herpes simplex) and ulceration
   Taste: postchemotherapy and tumor effect
   Esophagus: fungal infections, obstruction, and postradiation therapy inflammation
   Stomach: irritation and stasis
   Obstruction of the small bowel
   Constipation
Pancreatic carcinoma—gastric stasis
Hepatic metastases
Peritonitis
Central nervous system metastases
   Brain
   Meninges
Renal failure with uremia
Local infections and septicemia
Tumor toxins
Drugs
   Opioid analgesics
   Other medications such as digoxin and nonsteroidal anti-inflammatories
Radiation therapy, especially treatment of the gastrointestinal tract
Syndrome of cardiovascular autonomic insufficiency
Behavioral/psychogenic problems

Sources: Allan (1988); Bruera, Carrero, et al. (1986); Frytak and Moertel (1981).
[a]ADH, antidiuretic hormone.

patient with advanced metastatic liver disease on opioid analgesics. Therefore, the next step is the use of antiemetic drug therapy to control the symptoms.

The mechanism for controlling vomiting consists of two separate areas in the brain: the emetic center and the chemoreceptor trigger zone (CTZ) (Seigel and Longo 1981). The emetic center is the final common pathway that mediates all vomiting. In addition to input from the CTZ to the emetic center, the vestibular apparatus, the periphery (pharynx and gastrointestinal tract), and the cerebral cortex can in-

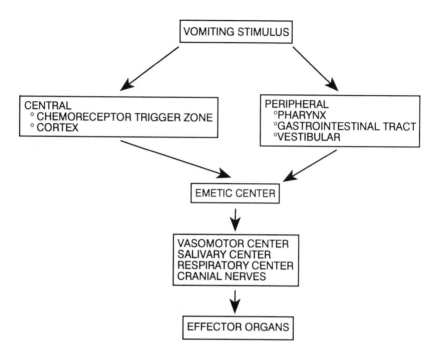

Figure 2.1   The Control Mechanism for Vomiting

duce emesis through the emetic center (fig. 2.1). Based on the extensive experience with the management of chemotherapy-induced nausea and vomiting, we can categorize antiemetic drugs as shown in table 2.2 (Siegel and Longo 1981; Dodds 1985).

Pharmacologic Treatment.   The pharmacologic treatment of patients with nausea and vomiting is similar in many aspects to that of patients with chronic pain, especially in regard to round-the-clock dosing and identifying patterns of the symptoms. It is difficult to generalize broadly based principles for the management of these patients because of the complexity of the problem. However, the following guidelines may be useful.

• The phenothiazines, such as prochlorperazine and thiethylperazine, are widely used antiemetic drugs and should be given initial consideration. Many of the phenothiazines as well as the antihistamines are available in liquid as well as suppository form.
• If nausea and vomiting are related to opioid analgesics such as morphine, antiemetic drugs can be added, similar to the use of

Table 2.2 Antiemetic Drugs for the Management of Nausea and Vomiting

Pharmacologic Classification	Example	Proposed Site(s) of Action	Usual Dose
Antihistamines	Diphenhydramine	? Emetic center/ cortex/vestibular	50–100 mg PO, IM, IV every 6–8h
Anticholinergic medications	Scopolamine	? Emetic center/ vestibular	Transdermal patch (0.5 mg) every 3 days
Dopamine antagonists			
Phenothiazines	Prochlorperazine	CTZ	5–20 mg PO or IM every 4–6h
Butyrophenones	Haloperidol	CTZ	0.5–2 mg PO or IM every 4–12h
Benzamides	Metoclopramide	Periphery/CTZ	10–15 mg PO every 6h
Cannabinoids	Dronabinol (delta-9-tetrahyrocannabinol)	Cortex	5–10 mg/m^2 PO every 4–6h
Corticosteroids	Dexamethasone	?	10–20 mg IV × 1
Benzodiazepines	Lorazepam	Cortex	1–2 mg PO, IV every 6–8h
5-HT$_3$ antagonist	Ondansetron	Peripheral	0.15 mg/kg IV every 4h × 3

Sources: Dodds (1985); Marin, Ilanez, and Arribas (1990); Seigel and Longo (1981).
Note: CTZ, chemoreptor trigger zone; PO, per os; IM, intramuscular; IV, intravenous; 5-HT$_3$, serotonin receptor.

prochlorperzine with the Brompton mixture (Melzack, Mount, and Gordon 1979). However, clinicians should exercise care, since the antiemetic drugs may potentiate the side effects of the opioid analgesics.

- If the syndrome of cardiovascular autonomic insufficiency and gastroparesis is suspected, treatment with metoclopramide is appropriate, since this drug accelerates gastric emptying (Kris et al. 1985).
- Patients with a history of motion sickness seem to be more susceptible to nausea and vomiting (Dodds 1985) and, therefore, may benefit from drug therapy that acts at the vestibular center, such as the antihistamines or the anticholinergic drugs.
- Nausea and vomiting due to malignant intestinal obstruction are difficult to treat, but the use of continuous-infusion antiemetic drugs seems to offer some relief (Baines, Oliver, and Carter 1985).
- For recalcitrant, intractable cases, a trial of continuous-infusion metoclopramide may be worthwhile in view of Warrington et al.'s (1986) experience in controlling chemotherapy-induced nausea and vomiting with this technique.

Pharmacologic intervention infrequently causes adverse reactions, the most common being extrapyramidal. Holmes, Adams, and Fernandez (1987) reported the unusual occurrence of respiratory dyskinesia and akathisia after the use of the butyrophenone droperidol as an antiemetic. Both respiratory dyskinesia and akathisia are acute extrapyramidal reactions due to droperidol. Respiratory dyskinesia is characterized by difficulty breathing and a gasping sensation that is frequently misdiagnosed as agitation or anxiety. Both of these extrapyramidal reactions respond promptly to anticholinergic drugs.

Nonpharmacologic Treatment. The nonpharmacologic management of nausea and vomiting is even less well delineated, and again the bulk of experience is extrapolated from the chemotherapy literature. Behavioral modification such as systemic desensitization is not practical in view of the length of time necessary to complete the procedure. To minimize or control, to some degree, the nausea and vomiting, one may instruct the patient and the family to do the following (Hogan 1986).

- Use interventions that have helped relieve nausea and vomiting during pregnancy, illness, or times of stress. Often a particular food or beverage associated with a past positive experience may effectively relieve the nausea.
- Eat cold foods or foods served at room temperature, such as sandwiches, cottage cheese, cereals, and desserts. These foods are usually tolerated better than are warm or hot foods, since the odors of hot foods often aggravate the feeling of nausea.
- Use a clear liquid diet to reduce nausea. Liquids such as apple juice, cranberry juice, lemonade, fruit ades, broth, ginger ale, tea, or cola are usually well tolerated. They should be sipped slowly. Bland foods such as popsicles, gelatin, mashed potatoes, applesauce, sherbet, crackers, toast, and cottage cheese are also well tolerated.
- Experiment with sour foods, such as lemons, sour pickles, hard sour candy, or lemon sherbet. The mouth can be rinsed with a mixture of lemon juice and water if stomatitis is not present.
- Avoid sweet, fatty, highly salted, and spicy foods as well as foods with strong odors.
- Minimize stimuli such as sights, sounds, or smells that can initiate nausea (e.g., unpleasant odors, strong perfume, other persons who are nauseated or vomiting, or the smell of food being cooked).
- Obtain fresh air by having the patient sit near an open window or outside.

• Provide distraction. Enjoyable music, a favorite television program, electronic games, talking with others, and reading are examples of effective distractions. Describing a favorite place, one's home, or a person who is significant can also provide distraction.
• Use techniques such as relaxation response, with or without positive visual imagery.

Anorexia and Cachexia

Anorexia, or diminished appetite, is a common finding in patients with advanced cancer. One study (Curtis, Krech, and Walsh 1991) of 100 oncology patients identified anorexia in 55 percent of the patients. The symptom of anorexia itself inevitably leads to weight loss, which in turn accelerates a loss of tissue mass, resulting in cachexia. This vicious cycle of anorexia-weight loss-cachexia, often referred to as the anorexia-cachexia syndrome, is difficult to break and becomes self-perpetuating, resulting in the common clinical picture of the emaciated, malnourished, dying patient.

Over the past decade, much scientific interest and enthusiasm has been generated regarding this problem. In a large multicenter study, the Eastern Cooperative Oncology Group (ECOG) studied the prognostic effect of weight loss before chemotherapy in 3,047 patients enrolled in 12 chemotherapy protocols (Dewys et al. 1980). The frequency of weight loss ranged from 31 percent for favorable non-Hodgkin lymphoma to 87 percent for gastric carcinoma. The median survival was significantly shorter in nine protocols for patients with weight loss compared to patients with no weight loss. Chemotherapy response rates were lower in patients with weight loss, but only in breast cancer patients was this difference significant. In short, the ECOG study clearly delineated the importance of weight loss as a prognostic factor across many institutions.

CAUSES

As a result of this research endeavor, a better understanding of the pathophysiology of the anorexia-cachexia syndrome has evolved. It is apparent that the causes of this syndrome are multiple and frequently overlapping. Three major causative components have been identified: systemic effects of cancer, local effects of cancer, and treatment-related complications (Rivlin, Shils, and Sherlock 1983).

The systemic effect of cancer is a frequent occurrence in clinical practice. This remote effect of tumor is thought to be a paraneoplastic syndrome, in the sense that a tumor-associated substance is the causative agent(s). Elements of the anorexia-cachexia syndrome include weight loss, weakness, asthenia, anemia, and protein, lipid, and carbohydrate metabolism abnormalities. The patient with this syndrome develops a negative energy balance in which the food intake is inappropriately less than the energy output, resulting in the net effect of loss of body weight (Langstein and Norton 1991). It has been suggested that tumor necrosis factor (TNF) is one substance contributing to the development of cancer-associated cachexia. Animal studies provided strong circumstantial evidence linking TNF with this problem. However, conflicting results have been reported regarding the presence of TNF in the serum of randomly selected cancer patients. Socher et al. (1988) assayed TNF levels in serum from 19 patients who had weight losses ranging from 8 to 40 percent of their preillness weight. This weight loss was not attributable to anticancer therapy, gastrointestinal disorders, or other medical problems. The investigators detected no TNF in serum samples from the 19 patients studied. Despite copious research, no specific agent has been conclusively identified. It is most likely that multiple cytokines, such as TNF, interleukin-1, interleukin-6, and interferon gamma, will be implicated in an interrelated fashion (Langstein and Norton 1991).

The local effects of cancer are generally mechanical or obstructive, depending on the tumor site. For example, patients with head and neck cancer may have difficulty swallowing, and those with gastrointestinal cancers may experience dysphagia, early satiety, obstruction, and malabsorption.

Finally, problems arising from the treatment of cancer may contribute to the anorexia-cachexia syndrome. Radiation therapy, especially to the oropharyngeal area, to the lower neck and mediastinum, and to the abdomen and pelvis, may cause significant nutritional problems, which are generally self-limited in time. Surgical procedures such as intestinal resections or bypass procedures of the small and large bowel cause more longstanding and chronic nutritional problems. Chemotherapy, like radiation therapy, may cause short periods of nutritional impairment usually related to drug-induced nausea and vomiting. Uncontrolled pain as well as the use of opioids to control pain may worsen the anorexia-cachexia syndrome.

By the time a patient is terminally ill, the contribution of cancer therapy to the anorexia-cachexia syndrome is less significant than is either the systemic or the local effects of cancer. What is often perceived at this point as related to treatment is in reality the clinical consequences of unopposed tumor growth.

MANAGEMENT

The treatment of the anorexia-cachexia syndrome and related nutritional problems in dying patients is slowly improving. Certainly, the use of intensive parenteral or enteral hyperalimentation has little value in the dying patient. The American College of Physicians (1989) concluded that the routine use of parenteral nutrition for patients undergoing chemotherapy should be strongly discouraged, and, in deciding to use such therapy in individual patients whose malnutrition is judged to be life threatening, physicians should take into account the possibility of increased risk.

Until recently, there were few publications in the medical literature regarding drug therapy for the anorexia-cachexia syndrome. What was published was mostly anecdotal. Several recent reports have suggested possible roles for corticosteroids, megestrol acetate, and dronabinol.

Corticosteroids. Corticosteroids have been used widely for years to alleviate the symptoms of cachexia and weakness in cancer patients, but without sound, scientific backing. For example, Schell (1972) strongly advocated the widespread use of corticosteroids in patients dying with advanced cancer because it not only increased appetite and a sense of well-being but also reduced the inflammatory response and opioid requirements. In 1982, Derogatis and MacDonald, reporting for an American Cancer Society Workshop, suggested the performance of prospective clinical trials on the use of corticosteroids in dying patients. In addition, they rightly pointed out that corticosteroids may cause symptoms of weakness and delirium, which are also commonly seen in patients with advanced cancer.

One of the earliest controlled and randomized studies on the use of corticosteroids in patients with advanced cancer was reported in 1974 by Moertel et al. from the Mayo Clinic. They studied 116 patients with far-advanced gastrointestinal cancer as part of a controlled, double-blind study comparing oral dexamethasone, 0.75 mg and 1.5 mg four times daily, to placebo. Two weeks after the start of treatment, more than half of the patients (57 percent) treated with dexamethasone reported an improvement in appetite, and more than one-fourth (26 percent) reported improved strength. However, this improvement may have been in large measure a placebo effect, since a substantial proportion of patients treated with the inactive placebo compound also reported improvement. By the fourth week, much of the initial improvement of symptoms in the placebo-treated patients had lessened and the dexamethasone-treated patients showed a substantial and significant advantage. According to the authors, this improvement of symptoms was largely the result of dexamethasone-induced euphoria, as only three dexamethasone-treated patients had gained weight and only two noted an improvement in their performance status. Finally, the investigators concluded that corticosteroid therapy did produce some improvement of symptoms in preterminal cancer patients with little discernible price in terms of side effects.

In 1984, Willox et al. studied sixty-one patients complaining of poor appetite or weight loss. The study was a double-blind, cross-over trial involving oral prednisolone, 5 mg three times daily for two weeks and then for a third week when the dosage was reduced, versus placebo. Forty-one of the 61 patients were evaluable: 16 men and 25 women, with an age range of 27 to 80 (mean, 60) years. Prednisolone was found to be significantly better than placebo in improving appetite during the three weeks of the study. This improvement was also seen when patients who had been taking placebo crossed over to receive prednisolone. There was a major placebo effect in half of the patients regarding improvement in appetite, which the authors interpreted as confirming a psychologic basis for anorexia in some patients. Weight gain did not occur in either group of patients. When taking prednisolone, patients showed a trend toward increased food intake and a significant increase in well-being. Finally, none of the patients reported any side effects.

In a more complex study, Bruera et al. (1985) explored the efficacy of oral methylprednisolone in a prospective, randomized trial in terminally ill cancer patients. A 14-day, double-blind, cross-over protocol was used to test methylprednisolone, 16 mg twice daily, against placebo. Forty patients were entered on the study, and 31 were evaluable (12 men and 19 women, with a mean age of 51 years). The authors found that appetite increased in 24 patients (77 percent). However, they observed no change of nutritional status and no serious toxicity during the study. They concluded that a short course (two weeks) of methylprednisolone increased the comfort of severely symptomatic patients with advanced cancer.

More recently, Della Cuna, Pellegrini, and Piazzi (1989) reported the effectiveness of an eight-week course of 125 mg of intravenous methylprednisolone per day in improving the quality of life in patients with preterminal cancer. This was a double-blind, placebo-controlled, multicenter study. Quality of life was assessed by several instruments. A total of 403 patients were enrolled in the study, with 207 being treated with methylprednisolone and 196 receiving placebo. Overall, methylprednisolone was significantly more effective than placebo in improving the quality of life, as judged by the changes from baseline in the quality-of-life scales. Although an improvement in appetite was reported more frequently in the methylprednisolone group, there was no significant difference between this treatment and placebo in regard to body weight changes.

In a second and related study, Popiela, Lucchi, and Giongo (1989) treated 173 terminally ill female cancer patients with either methylprednisolone or placebo. The methylprednisolone, at a dosage of 125 mg/day, was administered intravenously for eight consecutive weeks. Data were collected relative to the quality of life and other parameters. Eighty-five and 88 patients were randomized to treatment with methylprednisolone and placebo, respectively. As in the prior study, appetite showed consistent, often statistically significant, improvement across time in the methylprednisolone patients compared to the placebo group. However, this study did not monitor changes in weight.

Megestrol Acetate. Megestrol acetate is an oral progestational agent generally used in a dosage of 160 mg/day for diseases such as metastatic breast, endometrial, and renal cancer. It is well tolerated by patients except for occasional weight gain. Preliminary information suggested that megestrol acetate stimulates appetite and leads to nonfluid weight gain in some patients with metastatic breast and other cancers as well as in those with acquired immunodeficiency syndrome.

As part of a phase I and II trial studying the use of megestrol acetate in high dose as a treatment for breast cancer, Tchekmedyian et al. (1987) noted the presence of improved appetite and marked weight gain in these patients. The authors subsequently analyzed the pattern of weight change and the relationships of different variables to this weight change in those 28 patients with metastatic breast cancer treated with oral megestrol acetate (480 to 1,600 mg daily). Marked weight gain, ranging from 2 to 44 lb, was noted, and appetite enhancement was found in 96 percent of the patients. Weight gain occurred regardless of the pretreatment weight, extent of metastases, or response to therapy. Although these results were preliminary, the authors suggested a possible role for megestrol acetate in reversing anorexia and weight loss, thus improving the quality of life of patients with cachexia.

Loprinzi et al. (1990) studied 133 patients with advanced, incurable cancer treated with either megestrol acetate or placebo. Entry into this randomized, double-blind, placebo-controlled trial required that each patient must have lost at least 5 lb during the preceding two months or less and/or have had an estimated daily calorie intake of less than 20 Kcal/kg. Also, the attending physician must have determined that weight gain would have been beneficial to the patient. This multicenter, cooperative study (the North Central Cancer Treatment Group and the Mayo Clinic) included adult patients with advanced cancer except those with breast or endometrial sites. Before randomization, patients were stratified by primary site of disease, severity of weight loss, sex, and treatment with concurrent chemotherapy. Patients randomized to the megestrol acetate arm received 800 mg daily in three divided doses. The investigators collected extensive information, including a patient questionnaire.

In the group treated with megestrol acetate, 11 of 67 (16 percent) gained at least 15 lb, with 3 patients gaining more than 30 lb. Only one (2 percent) of the 66 patients treated with placebo gained this much. This difference was highly significant statistically. Of the patients in the megestrol acetate group, 16 percent gained 10 percent or more of their baseline weight, whereas no patients receiving placebo gained as much. There were no indications that the weight gain in these patients was related to the accumulation of excess fluid, such as ascites, edema, or pleural effusions. In those patients receiving concurrent chemotherapy, tumor regressions were not responsible for most of the weight gain seen in the study.

The investigators assessed the possibility of interaction between study treatment and each of the following factors: sex, age, primary tumor site, entry weight loss, performance status, and concurrent chemotherapy. They discovered no statistically significant interactions.

Toxicities were closely monitored. Patients in the megestrol acetate group experienced less nausea and emesis than did patients in the placebo group. Edema occurred more often in patients randomized to megestrol acetate (29 versus 13 percent), but clinically it was usually minimal and promptly responded to treatment with mild diuretics. Other possible side effects from megestrol acetate, such as impotence, irregular menses, and hypertension, were infrequent. No thrombotic events were noted in the patients receiving megestrol acetate. On the questionnaire, patients in the megestrol acetate group reported significantly better results for all questions related to appetite than did those assigned the placebo.

The authors thought that this study convincingly confirms that megestrol acetate can improve the appetite of patients with anorexia and cachexia associated with cancer and leads to substantial weight gain in some of these patients. Surprisingly, the study found an impressive and statistically significant reduction in nausea (38 versus 13 percent) and vomiting (25 versus 8 percent) in patients assigned to receive megestrol acetate. The authors speculated that megestrol acetate stimulates appetite, which in turn reduces the nausea and vomiting attributable to advanced malignant disease.

The optimal dose of megestrol acetate to stimulate appetite in patients with advanced cancer has not been determined. Prior studies in women with breast cancer suggest that there is a dose-response effect, and current research is ongoing in this area. Loprinzi et al. (1990) noted that treatment with 800 mg of megestrol acetate per day costs approximately $15 to $20 per day. Also unanswered is whether reversal of the anorexia and cachexia associated with advanced cancer will ultimately improve patient survival. In an updated study, Loprinzi et al. (1992) reported the results of a second North Central Cancer Treatment Group and Mayo Clinic trial, comparing three doses of megestrol acetate in patients with advanced cancer. A total of 343 eligible patients who had lost at least 5 lb in the previous two months or had a caloric intake of less than 20 Kcal/kg were randomized to receive megestrol acetate dosages of 160 mg/day (88 patients), 480 mg/day (86 patients), 800 mg/day (85 patients), or 1,280 mg/day (84 patients). Treatment groups were well balanced for prognostic factors. A positive dose-response effect on the patients' appetite and food intake was observed as the dosage of megestrol acetate increased from 160 mg/day to 800 mg/day. The data did not provide any support for dosages greater than 800 mg/day.

To elucidate further the mechanism of action of megestrol acetate, Reitmeier and Hartenstein (1990) treated 24 patients with this drug in dosages of 160 or 480 mg/day. All of these patients had advanced cancer of varying primary sites; they were anorectic and had sustained severe weight loss before treatment with megestrol acetate. Body composition was determined by measuring bioelectrical impedance. Analysis with this technique showed a shift from fat to lean body mass in patients with unchanged weight, whereas patients with weight gain had an increase of both fat and lean body mass. As noted by the authors, weight gain due to treatment with megestrol acetate was caused by an increase in fat and body cell mass and was not due only to fluid accumulation.

Cachexia is a common problem in patients infected with the human immunodeficiency virus (HIV) and is indicative of a poor prognosis. Von Roenn et al. (1988) treated 14 patients with megestrol acetate if they were HIV positive, had lost more than 10 percent of their preillness body weight, and were losing weight at the time of enrollment in the study. Patients were given megestrol acetate in a dosage of 80 mg four times a day (total daily dose of 320 mg). All patients gained weight at an average rate of approximately 1.1 lb/week. The average weight gain for the entire group was 14 lb. Therapy with megestrol acetate was well tolerated. Peripheral edema, thromboembolism, and impotence did not occur. All patients reported a significant improvement in appetite while on therapy. In addition, 7 patients reported a marked improvement in their sense of well-being. Although appetite improvement and weight gain in this study were encouraging, the true benefit of megestrol acetate for HIV-related cachexia and its effects on the quality of life need further assessment in the setting of a placebo-controlled trial.

A precautionary note on the use of megestrol acetate for AIDS-related cachexia was sounded by Henry et al. (1992). These investigators reported the development of insulin-dependent diabetes mellitus in a patient with AIDS 13 weeks after starting 320 mg of megestrol per day. When rechallenged with megestrol, the patient experienced an exacerbation of the diabetes. Until more information is available, the authors urged clinicians who manage patients with AIDS to be aware that megestrol acetate can induce a severe but reversible diabetic state and to use particular caution in patients with a predisposition for pancreatitis or diabetes.

Dronabinol. Interest has been renewed in the use of dronabinol (delta-9-tetrahydrocannabinol) as an appetite stimulant in patients with cancer. Wadleigh et al. (1990) studied 30 patients with unresectable cancer treated with oral dronabinol (delta-9-tetrahydrocannabinol in sesame oil). After a baseline observation period, patients were given dronabinol for up to six weeks at dosages of 2.5 mg once daily, 2.5 mg twice daily, or 5 mg once daily. Weekly weights were obtained, and each patient assessed appetite and mood on a visual analog scale. Five patients discontinued dronabinol because of adverse effects, and three stopped the drug due to progressive disease. Patients at all dosages continued to lose weight, although the rate of weight loss decreased with treatment at all dosages. Overall, improvement of symptoms was noted in both mood and appetite, with the dosage of 2.5 mg once daily being a no-effect dosage. Although the preliminary data are encouraging, more research is needed to delineate the role of this drug in the management of anorexia and cachexia.

Nutritional Problems

Many patients with advanced cancer and other diseases experience alterations in taste perceptions, especially a reduction in the pleasant taste of food and a bad taste sensation related to a specific food. This change in food taste in turn leads to a lessened appetite and a decreased caloric intake. Negative taste sensations are most often associated with meat, coffee, and chocolates (Dewys and Hoffman 1984).

Changes in taste only compound the anorexia and cachexia syndrome. Therefore, the goal of nutritional therapy at this stage is to

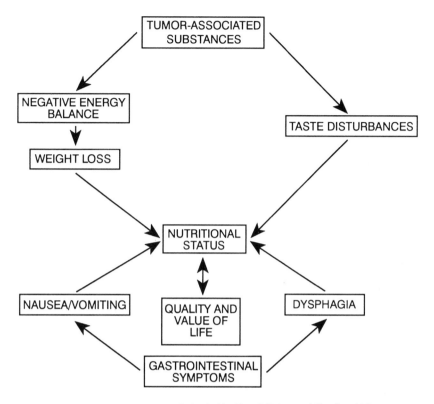

Figure 2.2   Factors Influencing a Patient's Nutritional Status and Quality of Life

improve the quality and value of life (fig. 2.2). With or without phar-macologic intervention, the patient is allowed to eat whatever and whenever he or she desires. Because of the emotional connotation of food, families need to be reassured that dying patients want only enough food and drink to keep them comfortable. Attempts to feed terminally ill patients artificially, particularly by the insertion of a na-sogastric tube, are likely to add to distress rather than relieve it (Ashby and Stoffell 1991).

Hydration

The issue of hydration in the dying patient is less clear and more controversial than that of nutrition (table 2.3). For example, in the Letters to the Editor section of *Lancet*, Waller, Adunski, and Hersh-kowitz (1991) reported their experience with the hydration of patients

Table 2.3   Pros and Cons in the Use of Hydration in Terminally Ill Patients

---

Pro

Dehydration and electrolyte imbalance may cause confusion, restlessness, and neuro-muscular irritability.

Dying patients are more comfortable if they receive hydration.

There is no evidence that fluids alone may prolong life.

Water is given to dying patients complaining of thirst, so why not administer paren-teral fluids?

Parenteral hydration is the minimum standard of care, and discontinuing this treat-ment breaks the bond with the patient.

Withholding fluids from dying patients is too close to the edge of withholding thera-pies from other compromised patients.

Con

Parenteral fluids may prolong the dying process.

Less urine output means less need for bedpan, urinal, commode, or catherization and fewer bed-wetting episodes.

There is less gastrointestinal secretion with fewer bouts of vomiting.

There is less salivary gland fluid with diminished salivation and drooling.

Less pulmonary secretion means less coughing, choking, pulmonary congestion, and death rattle.

Edema and ascites are minimized.

Diminished fluids and raised serum electrolyte levels may serve as a natural anesthetic to lessen the patient's level of consciousness.

It is normal and more comfortable to die dehydrated.

Sources: Fainsinger and Bruera (1991); Lamerton (1991); Zerwekh (1987).

dying within 48 hours. They compared two groups of 68 terminally ill cancer patients. One group of 13 patients (19 percent) received intra-venous (IV) fluids, while the second group was not given this treat-ment. The 19 percent of patients receiving IV fluids were treated at the request of their families. Blood urea nitrogen (BUN) and electrolyte levels were measured. BUN concentrations did not differ between patients receiving or not receiving IV fluids. However, serum sodium levels were significantly lower in the IV-treated patients. Also, there was a significant association between the state of consciousness and serum sodium values, although the level of consciousness did not cor-relate with the administration of IV fluids. The investigators con-cluded that, since most of their patients had severe hydration and electrolyte imbalance, including those receiving IV fluids, decisions about treatment with IV fluids should be based on the preference of the patient and family. This report by Waller, Adunski, and Hersh-kowitz (1991) elicited a sharp rebuff from Lamerton (1991) several weeks later. Lamerton argued that, if patients are hydrated before death, their bladders fill (causing urinary incontinence or distressing restlessness), their salivary glands produce excessive secretions and drooling, and their failing hearts become overloaded (causing dyspnea and worsening the death rattle). Furthermore, Lamerton (1991) thought that, although electrolytes and IV therapy might impress the family, it is normal and more comfortable to die slightly dehydrated.

Zerwekh (1987), working as a hospice nurse, reported her observations of the beneficial effect of dehydration in the dying patient. She noted that with dehydration there was decreased urine output, which resulted in less need for the bedpan, urinal, commode, or catherization and fewer episodes of bed-wetting. Gastrointestinal fluids were diminished, with fewer bouts of vomiting. Reduction in pulmonary secretions, with less coughing and pulmonary congestion, was observed. As pulmonary secretions were diminished, patients who had difficulty swallowing experienced relief from choking and drowning sensations. Zerwekh also reported that reduced fluids and increased serum electrolytes served as a natural anesthesia to lessen the patient's level of consciousness. The opposite effects were seen in patients who died while receiving IV fluids. Finally, the major symptoms of dehydration were thirst and dry mouth, both of which were managed by small sips of oral fluids and good oral care.

In 1989, Andrews and Levine reported the results of a mail survey of hospice nurses in New Jersey and Pennsylvania. The questionnaire consisted of two major sections. The first section was related to experience and asked if the nurses had observed any patient in whom no food or fluid was given or taken for at least three days before death. The second section was a series of statements about dehydration to which the respondants were asked to rate their agreement on a five-point scale. Ninety-six of the 127 questionnaires were completed and returned, for a 76 percent response rate. Overall, the study showed that hospice nurses who were experienced in the matter of terminal dehydration viewed it as beneficial in the terminal stages of life. It was found that with dehydration there was a diminution of distressing symptoms such as choking, vomiting, and drowning sensations. Finally, hospice nurses reported that aggressive nutritional and hydration therapies were not essential to keep dying patients comfortable.

The perception expressed by nurses that terminal dehydration abates some distressing symptoms is not uniformly shared by physicians. In a survey of physicians in the United States, three-fourths would have used intravenous fluids at a sufficient rate to maintain hydration in a theoretical case of a comatose dying patient. In this case, only one-fourth would have opted for a judicious amount of fluid or no intravenous infusion. Half of the physicians mentioned IV fluids as part of the standard care of dying patient. Thus, the use of intravenous fluids was often seen as "normal" in the terminal patient rather than as an extraordinary procedure for the treatment of hypercalcemia, hypoglycemia, and the like (Editorial, Terminal dehydration, 1986).

Finally, Fainsinger and Bruera (1991) advocated the use of hypodermoclysis (HDC) as an alternative to IV fluids for the dehydrated dying patient. HDC means the infusion of fluids into the subcutaneous space and offers many advantages over the intravenous route.

- Finding a venous access is unnecessary.
- HDC can be started by any staff member able to give a subcutaneous injection.
- HDC can be started and stopped without the needle clotting.
- Subcutaneous sites often last for days.

These investigators (Bruera et al. 1990) treated 58 patients with advanced cancer who required parenteral nutrition with HDC. There were 21 men and 37 women, with a mean age of 62 years. The reason for starting HDC was intestinal obstruction in 28 cases, nausea and vomiting in 10 cases, confusion in 14 cases, and dysphagia in 6 cases. HDC was administered using a no. 25 butterfly needle inserted underneath the skin of the anterior chest or abdominal wall. The needle was not changed until the site became symptomatic with pain, swelling, redness, or bleeding. A solution of two-thirds 5 percent dextrose and one-third saline was given at rates between 20 and 100 ml/hour. A total of 750 units of hyaluronidase, an enzyme that depolymerizes hyaluronic acid, causing a rapid diffusion of fluids subcutaneously, was added to each liter of solution. In addition, 20 to 40 mEq of potassium chloride per liter was mixed in the solution, and in 38 cases morphine or hydromorphone was administered as well. The mean duration of infusion was 14 ± 9 days, with a mean volume of 1.3 ± 0.8 L/day. The mean dose of potassium chloride was 25 ± 8 mEq/L. HDC was discontinued because of death in 43 patients, oral hydration in 12 patients, and a need for fluid restriction in 3 patients. Side effects were minimal: local infection (2 patients) and bruising (2 patients).

Constipation

Constipation is a common and often distressing symptom in patients with advanced disease. Although its cause varies, constipation is generally associated with abdominal pain and discomfort, poor appetite, and ultimately impaired nutritional status.

NARCOTIC BOWEL SYNDROME

Drugs such as opioid analgesics, anticholinergics, and antidiarrheal agents may produce constipation. In 1984, Sandgren, Mcphee, and Greenberger described the narcotic bowel syndrome (NBS) associated with the prolonged use or abuse of opioid analgesics in five patients. Clinical features of the NBS included chronic abdominal pain, nausea and vomiting, abdominal distension, constipation, and at least one episode of intestinal pseudo-obstruction. These symptoms rapidly resolved in all patients when the administration of opioids was stopped.

Opioid analgesics affect gastrointestinal function through sigma receptors for muscle tone located throughout the gastrointestinal tract. Opioids reduce gastrointestinal motility, with an increase in muscle tone in the gastric atrium and the first part of the duodenum. Gastric emptying is significantly delayed. Intestinal propulsive peristalsis is decreased while contractility and sphincter tone are enhanced. Lowered colonic motility as a result of opioids causes desiccated feces and constipation. Finally, opioids reduce gastric, biliary, and pancreatic secretions (Duthie and Nemmo 1987). Tolerance to the constipating effects of opioids often is absent or is slow to develop.

In an effort to delineate NBS in patients with advanced cancer, Bruera, Brenneis, Michaud, and MacDonald (1987) studied 191 patients treated with opioids between June 1985 and August 1986. All patients had metastatic disease without abdominal involvement, except 1 patient with liver metastases. Seven of the 191 (4 percent) were diagnosed as having NBS; all 7 had been receiving oral opioids, namely, morphine (3), hydromorphone (3) and levorphanol (1), for an average of 3 ± 2 months. The equivalent daily dose of oral morphine was 250 ± 170 mg. All patients developed severe bowel symptoms consistent with the diagnosis of NBS.

Hospitalization was required for management, including the use of parenteral analgesics. After metabolic abnormalities and mechanical intestinal obstruction were excluded, the patients were started on continuous subcutaneous infusions of metoclopramide (CISM) at a dosage of 60 mg/day using disposable portable pumps. Metoclopramide was chosen because it is known to increase gastrointestinal motility. Significant improvements in nausea, vomiting, appetite, and abdominal distension were observed in all patients within 72 hours of the start of the infusion. The patients were subsequently returned to oral opioids. The CISM was continued for 19 ± 6 days, with two patients being discharged home on this treatment. The CISM was discontinued because of unrelated death (one patient), return to oral metoclopramide (four patients), cessation of opioids (one patient), and toxicity (akathisia) after 14 days of infusion (one patient).

NONDRUG CAUSES

In addition to drugs such as opioid analgesics, there are other possible causes for constipation. Intestinal obstruction, be it malignant or benign, is one possibility. Indeed, in reporting the experience in managing intestinal obstruction at St. Christopher's Hospice in London, Baines, Oliver, and Carter (1985) found that 13 percent of patients with malignant intestinal obstruction had constipation. Metabolic disorders such as hypercalcemia, hypokalemia, and uremia may also cause constipation. Autonomic failure in the form of the syndrome of cardiovascular autonomic insufficiency is another cause for constipation (Bruera, Chadwick, Fox, et al. 1986). Occasionally a patient will present with constipation as one of the first signs of spinal cord or cauda equina compression from epidural metastases.

MANAGEMENT

After identifying and treating the underlying correctable causes, clinicians should encourage patients to increase their activity levels, especially ambulation, and oral intake of fluid. Barriers to defecation should be removed. Bedside commodes may be helpful for patients with limited ambulation. Most patients benefit from the addition of fiber to their diet. Excluding patients with intestinal obstruction, empiric therapy generally involves adding 3 to 4 grams of fiber to the daily diet and then gradually increasing this amount to 6 to 10 grams daily, as tolerated (Portenoy 1987).

Constipation may be prevented by anthraquinone cathartics (senna, cascara, danthron, and aloe). These drugs must undergo conversion to active metabolites in the colon and, therefore, are effective only in the distal colon. The anthraquinones act directly on the colon wall to stimulate peristalsis (Duthie and Nemmo 1987). Maguire, Yon, and Miller (1981) found that half a Senokot concentrated senna tablet (dose of 3.75 mg of total sennosides) reversed the constipating effect of 60 mg of codeine or its equivalent. For optimal results, the senna derivative was taken together with the analgesic or on a similar schedule.

In a randomized, cross-over clinical trial, Sykes (1991) compared a mixture of equal proportions of lactulose and senna to codanthramer (not available in the United States) standard strength in 117 cancer patients with constipation. Patients with bowel diversion and evidence of intestinal obstruction were excluded. The lactulose-senna mixture produced a significantly greater frequency of stool than did codanthramer in patients receiving morphine and reduced the usage of suppositories and enemas. The incidence of diarrhea was greater with lactulose-senna; however, this generally dissipated with a 24-hour break and usually did not recur with the next dose. The patients' subjective assessment indicated that lactulose-senna was more likely than codanthramer to relieve constipation or to restore normalcy. Because increased doses of laxative were needed as the opioid doses increased, Sykes (1991) suggested that a schedule of laxative doses in relation to opioid doses may improve the effectiveness of laxative therapy over a system of ad hoc titration from a starting dose. Finally, a direct relationship between laxative and opioid doses was not observed, implying that opioids became relatively less constipating as the dosage was raised.

Other management for constipation includes the use of rectal agents and oral laxatives. Rectal agents include suppositories and enemas. Suppositories may contain glycerin alone, drawing fluid into the rectum and acting as a stimulant to defecation, or may contain an active drug such as bisacodyl. Enemas with tap water, saline, or soap suds may be used. Both suppositories and enemas are useful for the treatment of acute constipation or for the management of fecal impaction.

Oral cathartics include bulk-forming laxatives, lubricants, and osmotic (saline) cathartics. Bulk-forming laxatives, like bran, psyllium, and methycellulose, increase the stool bulk and soften its consistency by increasing the mass and water content of the stool. These agents are generally effective after two to four days of daily use. Of the lubricants, oral mineral oil is the preferred substance. This agent lubricates the stool, allowing easier passage. In obtunded or confused patients, aspiration with a resultant lipoid pneumonia is a significant risk. This substance has little role in the management of chronic constipation but is useful in the acute treatment of fecal impaction or in acute transient constipation. Osmotic (saline) cathartics draw fluid into the bowel lumen, thereby decreasing the transit time of the stool. Magnesium salts, sodium salts, and lactulose are agents in this category. The use of magnesium and sodium salts is limited in patients with renal failure and congestive heart failure because of the systemic absorption of these ions. Generally, the magnesium and sodium salts are effective for rapid evacuation within three to six hours. Lactulose is more effective for chronic use in dosages ranging from 15 to 30 ml, two to four times a day.

The contact cathartics are the primary agents used in the management of chronic constipation. These drugs cause increased mucosal secretion and a change in gastrointestinal motility. The docusates, anthraquinone, and diphenylmethane derivatives, as well as castor oil, are included in this category. Dioctyl sulfosuccinate is a docusate that is widely available and is often added as a stool softener to other contact cathartics. The diphenylmethane derivatives phenolphthalein and bisacodyl produce effects similar to those of the anthraquinones. Generally, they are safe and well tolerated for the management of constipation. The last of the contact cathartics is castor oil, but this agent is seldom used except in the management of acute, self-limited constipation (Portenoy 1987).

CENTRAL NERVOUS SYSTEM SYMPTOMS

Delirium

Delirium (acute confusional states) has been known and described since Hippocrates. It has been called "everyone's psychosis" or "reversible madness" and is one of the most commonly encountered mental disorders in general hospital practice. Indeed, it is estimated that approximately 10 percent of hospitalized medical and surgical patients are delirious at any given time (Lipowski 1987). The reported incidence of delirium in patients dying with cancer ranges from 53 to 85 percent (Bruera, Chadwick, Weinlick, et al. 1987; Massie, Holland, and Glass 1983).

By definition, delirium is a transient disorder of cognition and attention, one accompanied by disturbances of the sleep-wake cycle and psychomotor activity. It is classified as one of the organic brain syndromes. Elderly patients are especially prone to delirium, and it has been associated with a high mortality. Self-injury of the patient is a serious risk, as are legal and ethical complications.

The cardinal clinical features of this syndrome are disorders of cognition and attention, disruption of the normal sleep-wake cycle, and either reduced or heightened activity and responsiveness. These symptoms develop acutely. They frequently fluctuate in severity during the day and are most pronounced at night.

Cognitive functions, mainly perception, thinking, and memory, are impaired to varying degrees. Disordered perception often results in confusion in addition to visual and auditory illusions. Thinking is disorganized and incoherent, which is evident in the patient's speech. Memory is impaired in all key aspects and orientation is usually defective, especially with regard to time. Attention (awareness, consciousness) is always disordered and attentional disturbances typically fluctuate during the day.

The normal sleep-wake cycle is disrupted. Often the patient sleeps or naps during the day, but at night he or she tends to be awake and agitated. This disorganized cycle seems to enhance the cognitive and attention deficits. Psychomotor behavior is altered in that the patient's movements and speech may be hypoactive or hyperactive. Hyperactivity is not a hallmark of delirium. Finally, emotions ranging from apathy or depression to fear or rage may also be present.

No specific diagnostic test for delirium is available, and the diagnosis is established on the basis of its essential clinical features. Cognitive and attentional symptoms are elicited and observed at the bedside. In general, the acute onset of cognitive and attention deficits and abnormalities, whose severity fluctuates during the day and tends to worsen at night, is practically diagnostic (Lipowski 1987).

Differentiating delirium from dementia is especially important and may be difficult when delirium is superimposed on preexisting dementia. A history of intellectual decline, occurring months or years before the onset of the acute cognitive disorder, is crucial for the differential diagnosis. In contrast to the delirious patient, the demented patient is usually alert and aware of the surroundings, fails to show fluctuating levels of awareness during the daytime, and shows defective knowledge of commonly known facts. The acute deterioration of cognitive and attentional functions in a known demented patient suggests delirium (Lipowski 1989).

CAUSES

The occurrence of delirium in cancer patients is related to a wide range of causative factors, all of which can lead to diffuse cerebral dysfunction. Posner (1979) classified the neurologic complications of systemic cancer into the following areas: metastases to the nervous system, nonmetastatic involvement through metabolic encephalopathy (related to vital organ failure, electrolyte imbalance, and nutritional abnormalities), infections, vascular disorders, side effects of therapy (including opioid analgesic use), and paraneoplastic syndromes. Subacute cerebellar degeneration, limbic encephalitis, and progressive multifocal leukoencephalopathy are types of remote effects of tumor or paraneoplastic syndromes that may present with dementia early in the course of the disease or may even precede the diagnosis of cancer. It is important, therefore, to recognize and diagnose these entities, since delirium may be superimposed on the process.

To understand better this syndrome of delirium in patients dying of cancer, Massie, Holland, and Glass (1983) studied 13 patients with cancer who died during their hospitalization. Eleven of the 13 (85 percent) developed delirium as measured by a standardized delirium scale. Typically, the delirium developed as the patient's illness progressed and appeared most frequently when the patient was near death. In 2 of the 11 patients it was not possible to discover the cause, since no laboratory tests were performed. In all of the remaining cases (9), delirium was attributed to metabolic encephalopathy, structural invasion of the brain by tumor, or a combination. Factors identified as causing the metabolic encephalopathy were the failure of a vital organ (such as kidney, liver, or lung), toxic levels of opioids, electrolyte imbalance, and sepsis. In more than half of the patients, the metabolic encephalopathy was due in part to increasing doses of opioid analgesics. In this study, it was difficult to establish a single cause for delirium in patients with advanced cancer.

In a less controlled study, Bruera, Chadwick, Weinlick, et al. (1987) retrospectively reviewed the cases of 30 consecutive patients who died after being admitted to the hospital for at least one week under their care. All the patients had metastatic cancer. Unlike the study by Massie, Holland, and Glass (1983), this study did not use a standardized delirium scale. The diagnosis of delirium was made clinically in the presence of a confusional state with or without hallucinations or hyperactivity. Sixteen of the 30 patients (53 percent) developed delirium, by the authors' definition, more than 48 hours before death. In only 2 of these cases (13 percent) was a cause found, and in both it was related to drug therapy (amitriptyline and morphine). Also, improvement was noted in both of these cases after either discontinuation or change in drug treatment.

Stedeford and Regnard (1991) provided a systematic scheme for assessing delirium in patients with advanced cancer (table 2.4). Reduced alertness is common in acute confusional states. Opioid analgesics are frequently blamed, but they are an unlikely cause in a patient receiving them chronically. Commonly overlooked drugs include corticosteroids, nonsteroidal anti-inflammatory drugs, and antidepressants. Infections, especially respiratory and urinary, may change alertness, as will metabolic alterations such as hypercalcemia, hyponatremia, and uremia. The presence of underlying cardiac or pulmonary disease may cause hypoxia accompanied by increased alertness and marked anxiety.

An unsuspected subdural hematoma or an impacted bone fracture may reduce alertness and cause confusion. Finally, abnormal experiences and hallucinations are infrequently related to the use of morphine. Tolerance to this side effect may occur.

Table 2.4   The Symptoms and Causes
of Delirium

Symptoms
   Memory failure
   Changed alertness
   Impaired concentration
   Abnormal experiences
   Altered behavior
   Mood disturbance

Causes
   Drugs
      Opioids
      Corticosteroids
      Antidepressants
      Nonsteroidal anti-inflammatories
   Infection
      Respiratory
      Urinary
   Metabolic disturbances
      Hypercalcemia
      Hyponatremia
      Uremia
   Cardiac or pulmonary disease
   Brain disease
      Metastases
   Trauma
      Subdural hematoma
      Impacted bone fracture
   Treatable anxiety or depression
   Unrelated psychiatric illness

Source: Stedeford and Regnard (1991).

MANAGEMENT

Once the diagnosis of delirium is made, the following guidelines
may be useful in the management of this syndrome (Levine, Silberfarb,
and Lipowski 1978; Lipowski 1987, 1989; Massie, Holland, and Glass
1983; Stedeford and Regnard 1991).

- If you suspect metabolic encephalopathy secondary to opioid analgesic use, change the opioid. Avoid polypharmacy, since drugs
other than opioids have also been implicated.
- Provide measures to help reduce anxiety, agitation, and disorientation. These may include a quiet, well-lit room with a few familiar
objects and a visible calendar and clock. Short but frequent contacts with a supportive person, preferably a family member, help

alleviate the disorientation. Good nursing care is crucial for orienting and reassuring the patient.

• The impaired ability to function mentally is very distressing to patients who are acutely aware of it. Depression, with possible suicidal risk, must be kept in mind because of the patient's poor impulse control.

• Sedation may be necessary to relieve severe agitation, disruptive behavior, or insomnia. Haloperidol is usually the safest and most effective drug for this purpose. Massie, Holland, and Glass (1983) suggested that the intramuscular injection of 0.5 to 2 mg reduces agitation without causing sedation or hypotension. Doses, repeated at 30- to 60-minute intervals, are then titrated against behavior. Extrapyramidal signs are controlled by benzotropine, 2 mg twice a day. The authors also recommended changing the patient to an oral dose as soon as possible, at three-quarters of the level of the intramuscular dose. For lesser degrees of disturbed behavior they suggested the use of 1 mg of haloperidol, 1 to 2 mg of trifluoperazine, or 10 to 25 mg of thioridazine given orally twice daily.

• Psychiatric involvement to help interpret the situation for the family and collaborate with the staff in the management of the patient is useful.

Depression

Psychologic problems, especially depression, are often assumed to be common in cancer patients. Despite the recent advances in the treatment of cancer, the diagnosis is still terrifying to patients and families. Their initial reaction is generally shock and denial. Patients may complain of feeling depressed, anxious, and irritable. They may experience a loss of appetite and insomnia during the first 7 to 10 days after the diagnosis. This acute stress response is considered normal and is usually resolved when treatment is started. For some patients, however, these symptoms persist and may interfere with medical management.

Diagnosis

Apart from the acute stress response, reactive depression is the most frequent psychologic problem diagnosed in patients with cancer (Holland 1987). Depending on the method of diagnosis used, the prevalence rate for depression in these patients seems to be between 23 and 58 percent (Brown et al. 1986). However, many of these studies were flawed by the use of biased samples or reliance on self-report instruments. In an effort to identify psychologic problems in cancer patients, the Psychosocial Collaborative Oncology Group (PSYCOG) studied 215 randomly accessed patients from three major cancer treatment centers (Derogatis et al. 1983). Each patient was evaluated by a common protocol comprising a formal psychiatric interview and standardized psychologic tests. The American Psychiatric Association's *Diagnostic and Statistical Manual of Mental Disorders* (DSM-III) was used in making the diagnosis. The prevalence rate of mental disorders among the cancer patients was high, at 47 percent.

The authors noted that this is about twice the rate usually found in medical patients and three times as high as prevalence rates reported for the general population. However, the most frequent diagnoses were adjustment disorders, which accounted for 68 percent of the psychiatric diagnoses. These adjustment disorders consisted of varying elements of anxiety and depression and were attributed to the stress of the diagnosis of cancer. Thirteen percent had a major depression, 8 percent had organic mental disorders related to analgesics or metabolic abnormalities, 7 percent had personality disorders that predated the illness, and 4 percent of those patients with a positive psychiatric condition were experiencing a disorder with depression or anxiety as the central symptom.

Another major finding of the PSYCOG study was that most of the psychiatric disorders found in the sample of cancer patients can be successfully treated. In addition, the fact that most (53 percent) of these patients did not have any psychiatric disorder revealed by a careful diagnostic interview should not be ignored. Despite the terror commonly associated with cancer, most patients are able to mobilize their psychologic resources in a normal, reasonably adaptive way (Glass 1983).

In a recent review, Cody (1990) suggested that adjustment disorders are common, observed in some 25 to 35 percent of patients. Only a small minority, approximately 5 to 15 percent, become seriously depressed, which, she felt, dispels the myth that depression is an inevitable reaction to a terminal illness.

Clinical symptoms, such as anorexia, weight loss, and fatigue, are common to both cancer and depression and therefore are of little value in diagnosing depression in the cancer patient. Thus, the diagnosis must rely heavily on psychologic symptoms, such as the presence of dysphoric mood (sadness, anxiety) and feelings of hopelessness, helplessness, and worthlessness. The differentiation between reactive depression and major depression is often difficult, as these two diagnoses represent a continuum of severity of depressive symptoms rather than two separate diagnostic categories.

Cancer patients at high risk for developing depression include those with poor pain control; a more deteriorated physical condition; advanced stages of disease, especially pancreatic cancer; and a history of prior depression or psychiatric illness (Holland 1987).

DEPRESSION AND SUICIDE

In 1986, Brown et al. studied 44 terminally ill patients from the palliative care service at St. Boniface General Hospital to determine whether suicidal thinking was a normal finding in dying patients. Among these 44 patients, the majority (34) had never wished death to come early. Of the remaining 10 patients, 3 were or had been suicidal and 7 more were suffering from clinical depressive illness. The authors thought that suicidal thoughts and desires for death seemed to be linked exclusively to the presence of a mental disorder. Furthermore, generalizing their findings, the authors postulated that patients with terminal illness who are not mentally ill are no more likely than the general population to wish for premature death.

In a related article, Breitbart (1987) reviewed the topic of suicide in cancer patients. Few systematic studies have been done to determine the true incidence of cancer suicide; however, these studies do suggest that, although relatively few cancer patients commit suicide, they are at increased risk. The frequency of passive suicide and the degree of treatment noncompliance or refusal, which represents a deliberate decision to end life, are unknown, and the actual incidence of suicide in cancer patients may be underestimated. Men with cancer are at increased risk of suicide compared to the general population. The most common method of suicide in the cancer patient is a medication overdose of either sleep or pain drugs. According to Breitbart, factors in the vulnerability to suicide with cancer are advanced illness and poor prognosis, delirium, loss of control and helplessness, preexisting psychopathology, prior and family suicide history, exhaustion, and fatigue.

MANAGEMENT

The treatment of depression may include short-term supportive psychotherapy and psychopharmacologic drugs. Short-term supportive psychotherapy is generally effective for patients with a normal response to stress or an adjustment disorder. This mode of treatment is based on a crisis intervention model, and 4 to 10 sessions are generally sufficient to reduce symptoms to a tolerable level. The inclusion of a family member or close friend in these sessions has been found to be helpful. Group sessions with patients who share the same problem are an alternative approach (Holland 1987).

Prolonged or severe symptoms indicate the presence of a major depression, which should be managed with a combined regimen of supportive psychotherapy and psychopharmacologic drugs.

The tricyclic antidepressants have been the mainstay in the treatment of depression (Cody 1990; Holland 1987). They are also useful in the management of neuropathic pain, which is independent of their effect on mood. Amitriptyline, imipramine, doxepin, and nortriptyline are most commonly prescribed. In cancer patients and patients with other terminal illnesses, treatment is generally empiric because of the paucity of good scientific data from randomized clinical trials.

The tricyclic antidepressants have generally equivalent clinical efficacy and differ only in the intensity of side effects (table 2.5). The choice of antidepressants is usually dictated by the patient's clinical state. Depressed patients with agitation, anxiety, and insomnia usually welcome the sedative properties of drugs such as amitriptyline, whereas patients with psychomotor retardation respond better to the activating drugs such as imipramine.

The main side effect of the tricyclic antidepressants is their effect on the cardiovascular system, namely, delay in cardiac conduction or arrhythmia (Potter, Rudorfer, and Manji 1991), and orthostatic hypotension. Anticholinergic side effects are often bothersome, especially dry mouth, blurred vision, hesitancy of micturition, urinary retention, and

Table 2.5   The Side Effects of Antidepressant Drugs

Drug	Sedation	Insomnia	Anticholinergic Effects	Orthostatic Hypotension	Nausea	Usual Daily Oral Dose (mg)
Tricyclic drugs						
Amitriptyline	+++	0	+++	++	0	75–150
Imipramine	++	0	+++	+++	0	75–150
Doxepin	+++	0	++	+++	0	75–150
Nortriptyline	++	0	+	+	0	100–150
Newer drugs						
Trazodone	+++	0	+	++	+	150–250
Maprotiline	++	0	+	++	0	50–75
Amoxapine	++	0	+	++	0	100–150
Alprazolam	+	0	0	0	0	1.5

Sources: Cody (1990); Potter, Rudorfer, and Manji (1991); Holland (1987).

Note: 0 = no side effect; + = minor side effect; ++ = moderate side effect; +++ = major side effect.

constipation. Patients already receiving opioids may experience a worsening of dry mouth and constipation. Over time, a tolerance to these unwanted side effects seems to develop (Cody 1990).

For poorly understood reasons, patients with cancer or other chronic disease seem to respond to lower doses than do otherwise physically normal patients. In practice, it is best to tailor the dose to the response and the severity of side effects. Amitriptyline, for example, is started at 10 to 20 mg/day given at bedtime and increased by 25 mg every one or two days until a beneficial effect occurs. Generally, all antidepressants take two to three weeks to exert their antidepressant effect, although patients may benefit from the anxiolytic or sedative effect much earlier.

The second-generation antidepressants (trazodone, maprotiline, amoxapine, and alprazolam) should be considered for patients not responding to the tricyclic antidepressants or for those who cannot tolerate the side effects of anticholinergic drugs. This new generation of drugs, however, has not been shown to be superior to the tricyclic antidepressants in terms of antidepressant effects.

In one of the few randomized clinical trials, Holland et al. (1991) compared alprazolam to progressive muscle relaxation in cancer patients with anxiety and depressive symptoms. One hundred forty-seven cancer patients were randomized to receive either alprazolam, 0.5 mg three times a day, or a progressive muscle relaxation technique over a 10-day period. Seventy patients were randomized to drug and 77 to relaxation. Four measures of anxiety and depression were utilized. Both treatment arms resulted in a significant decrease in observer- and patient-reported anxious and depressed symptoms. Although both treatments were effective, patients receiving alprazolam showed a slightly more rapid decrease in anxiety and a greater reduction of depressive symptoms. Based on their study, the investigators recommended the use of alprazolam and relaxation in cancer patients experiencing symptoms of anxiety and depression.

Finally, antidepressants of the monoamine oxidase inhibitor class are unsuitable for depressed cancer and terminally ill patients because of the necessity for dietary restrictions (Cody 1990).

SYSTEMIC SYMPTOMS

Dyspnea

Dyspnea, or shortness of breath, is a distressing symptom to both the patient and the family. In 1974, Wilkes reported dyspnea as one of the

10 major symptoms after admission to a small 25-bed unit especially interested in caring for the dying patient. Reuben and Mor, in 1986, reviewed the epidemiology of dyspnea in terminal cancer patients during the last six weeks of life. This study found dyspnea to be more common in these patients (70.2 percent) than had previously been appreciated. In addition, the severity of the symptom was at least moderate in more than 28 percent of patients who were able to grade their dyspnea (Reuben and Mor 1986a). In 1989, Higginson and McCarthy reported that, near death, 21 percent of their patients developed dyspnea as the main symptom. Furthermore, this became the most common severe symptom at death.

DYSPNEA WITH MALIGNANT DISEASE

Lung cancer is the leading cause of cancer death in men and women in the United States. Therefore, it is not surprising that the presence of this disease correlates highly with the symptom of dyspnea. The pathophysiology producing shortness of breath in patients with lung cancer includes

- endobronchial or central lesions causing obstruction resulting in atelectasis or pneumonia;
- parenchymal replacement by tumor to the extent that a restrictive ventilatory defect occurs;
- diffuse lymphangitic spread of the tumor throughout the lungs;
- phrenic nerve paralysis from compression by mediastinal lymph node metastases leading to impaired diaphragmatic function;
- pleural effusions resulting in reduced lung capacity; and
- superior vena caval syndrome.

Dyspnea may occur by differing mechanisms in patients with pulmonary metastases. For example, the sudden onset of shortness of breath in patients with known parenchymal disease suggests the development of an associated effusion, bleeding into a metastasis with sudden subpleural expansion, or the occurrence of a pneumothorax. Likewise, the onset of increasing dyspnea associated with cough and debilitation often denotes lymphangitic carcinomatosis despite a normal chest radiograph (Pass and Roth 1987). Thus, like pain, dyspnea must be evaluated on an ongoing periodic basis to monitor any changes, be they subtle or obvious.

Finally, other factors can cause or contribute to the clinical symptom of dyspnea, such as

- prior cancer treatment with surgery (postpneumonectomy), radiation therapy (postradiation pulmonary fibrosis), or chemotherapy (the use of bleomycin, for example);
- generalized debility of terminal disease;
- pulmonary embolism;
- aspiration pneumonia;
- the presence of underlying disease, especially chronic obstructive pulmonary disease and congestive heart failure;
- massive ascites compromising pulmonary function; and
- anxiety, which frequently can enhance dyspnea during breathless attacks (Higginson and McCarthy 1989) (table 2.6).

DYSPNEA WITH NONMALIGNANT DISEASES

Nonmalignant advanced diseases can cause dyspnea (table 2.7). Chronic progressive cardiac and respiratory diseases frequently end with terminal dyspnea. Aspiration pneumonia is often missed as a cause of shortness of breath, as it may occur silently during sleep in

Table 2.6   The Causes of Dyspnea in Patients
with Advanced Cancer

Carcinoma of the lung
  Obstructing lesions with atelectasis and pneumonia
  Restrictive ventilatory defect
  Lymphangitic spread
  Metastases
  Impaired diaphragmatic function
  Pleural effusions
  Superior vena caval syndrome
  Bleeding
  Pneumothorax
Prior cancer therapy
  Postpneumonectomy
  Postradiation fibrosis
  Chemotherapy
Generalized debility
Thrombotic pulmonary embolism
Tumor pulmonary embolism
Aspiration pneumonia
Pneumonia due to infection
Underlying chronic obstructive pulmonary disease or congestive
    heart failure
Massive ascites
Anxiety

Sources: Pass and Roth (1987); Higginson and McCarthy (1989).

Table 2.7   The Causes of Dyspnea
in Patients with Advanced
Nonmalignant Disease

Chronic obstructive pulmonary disease
Congestive heart failure
Infection
Chronic congestive heart failure
Aspiration pneumonia
Recurrent pulmonary embolism
Chest wall deformity
Intercostal or diaphragmatic weakness
Anemia
Drugs

Source: Regnard and Ahmedzai (1991).

conditions in which esophagopharyngeal muscle tone is impaired, as in motor neuron disease or systemic sclerosis. Deformity of the chest wall causing dyspnea may be the consequence of prior poliomyelitis, kyphoscoliosis, or ankylosing spondylitis. Chronic intercostal or diaphragmatic weakness may result from motor neuron disease. Finally, the chronic use of drugs can cause dyspnea through diffuse lung injury (Regnard and Ahmedzai 1991).

MANAGEMENT

As with the management of pain and other symptoms in the dying patient, the clinician should seek causes for dyspnea and, when these are identified, take corrective action. For example, bronchodilators can be helpful in relieving symptomatic bronchospasm. Saunders (1982) outlined a group of drugs useful in the management of dyspnea. Corticosteroids may be used in the management of mediastinal lymph node compression resulting from superior vena caval obstruction, lymphangitic carcinomatosis of the lung, and bronchospasm. Antibiotics are recommended on an individual basis rather than being administered routinely. Factors such as the symptoms caused by the pneumonia and the patient's age, overall condition, and respiratory capacity should be considered. If antibiotics are not justified, then symptoms can be controlled by the use of opioids and anticholenergic medications such as scopolamine. In a study (Volicer et al. 1986) of 40 patients with Alzheimer disease, 62 percent were not treated with antibiotics if they developed symptoms of pneumonia. The authors of the study thought that the treatment of infections with antibiotics did not necessarily increase patients' comfort. Furthermore, the authors did not favor empiric antibiotic therapy without a work-up and stated that the patients' comfort was maintained by the frequent use of analgesics and antipyretics.

Small doses (5 to 10 mg every four hours) of morphine effectively relieve dyspnea. Morphine is known to decrease the ventilatory response to carbon dioxide, hypoxia, and exercise and to diminish oxygen consumption at rest and during exercise in normal persons. Morphine also reduces the respiratory rate and the sensation of gasping for air or air hunger (Cooke 1989). As with pain control, the clinician should titrate the dose against the response and increase it as needed. Tranquilizers, such as chlorpromazine or diazepam, may be added to manage the anxiety associated with dyspnea. Hoskin and Hanks (1988) reported their experience with advanced cancer patients admitted to the Continuing Care Unit at the Royal Marsden Hospital. They found that the prime indication for morphine in 22 percent of the patients was for the relief of respiratory symptoms rather than pain.

A small bedside fan is often effective in managing terminal dyspnea (Kerr 1989). Preferably, the fan is placed to propel fresh air from an open window across the patient's face. This stream of cool air stimulates temperature and mechanical receptors of the facial trigeminal nerve in the cheek, thus altering the perception of breathlessness. Trigeminal nerve receptors also line the nasopharynx, and this may explain why some patients experience relief of dyspnea from the use of nasal oxygen.

The accumulation of excessive pulmonary secretions when the patient is dying, the so-called death rattle, is quite disturbing for families and staff. Generally, this can be managed with scopolamine in doses of 0.4 to 0.6 mg given every four to eight hours as required (Cooke 1989; Saunders 1982). Saunders (1982) also recommended administering concomitant morphine, 10 to 15 mg, to increase sedation and prevent the occasional central nervous system excitement caused by scopolamine. In the study by Hoskin and Hanks (1988), scopolamine by injection was given with diamorphine to ameliorate respiratory symptoms from retained pulmonary secretion in 34 percent of their patients. One patient received a four-day infusion. When scopolamine was administered by injection, the median number of injections required was 1, with a mean of 3.6 and a range of 1 to 20.

Saunders (1982) suggested that oxygen can be useful in acute dyspnea but that better control of chronic dyspnea can be achieved with opioids. Supplemental oxygen should be used with care in patients with chronic obstructive pulmonary disease, who may retain carbon dioxide. Kerr (1989), however, questioned the necessity of using oxygen in the dyspneic dying patient. He pointed out the occurrence of a bedside medical melodrama with all attention focused on the oxygen, its flow rate, and the placement of the cannula.

In patients with large pleural effusions, rapid relief of dyspnea occurs after the removal of the pleural fluid. Evidence suggests that this improvement in breathing is due to a reduction in the thoracic cage size, which allows the inspiratory muscles to operate more efficiently (Estenne, Yernault, and DeTroyer 1983). Thus, in the dyspneic patient with a pleural effusion, a therapeutic thoracocentesis is reasonable and may result in clinical improvement.

Finally, coughing often accompanies the shortness of breath. Expectorants, which increase the volume of sputum, are generally not helpful. Mucolytic drugs, such as acetylcysteine, reduce the viscosity of bronchial secretions and occasionally are useful. In patients on opioid analgesics for pain control, escalating the dose is often effective in suppressing the cough as well.

Given this array of therapeutic interventions for the management of dyspnea, it is quite interesting that Higginson and McCarthy (1989) concluded from their study that these treatments are generally ineffective. Utilizing a standardized measurement instrument, symptom assessment scores for patients with dyspnea showed no change over time despite a variety of treatments. According to the authors, uncontrolled dyspnea should receive more research attention.

Urinary Incontinence

The involuntary loss of urine or urinary incontinence is a clinical problem that has often been overlooked and is poorly understood. In a study by Wilkes (1974) more than 15 years ago, incontinence was one of the 10 major symptoms after admission in 296 patients cared for in a small, 25-bed palliative care unit in England. In this same study, urinary incontinence was the reason for admission to respite care in 11 percent of the cases.

As reviewed by the Consensus Conference on Urinary Incontinence in Adults (1989), continence requires a compliant bladder and active sphincteric mechanisms such that maximum urethral pressure always exceeds intravesical pressure. Normally, voiding requires sustained and coordinated relaxation of the sphincters and contraction of the urinary bladder. These functions are regulated by the central nervous system through both autonomic and somatic nerves. This system requires the integration of visceral and somatic muscle function and involves control by voluntary mechanisms originating in the cerebral cortex. These voluntary mechanisms are learned and culturally pre-scribed (that is, toilet training).

CAUSES

Incontinence can be produced by any pathologic, anatomic, or phys-iologic factor that disrupts the pressure gradient between the bladder and the urethra. In the general adult population, the most common clinical forms of urinary incontinence are stress incontinence, urge incontinence, overflow incontinence, and a mixed form. In stress in-continence, dysfunction of the bladder outlet causes a leakage of urine as intraabdominal pressure is raised above urethral resistance while coughing, bending, or lifting heavy objects. Stress incontinence has many causes, including direct anatomic damage to the urethral sphinc-ter.

Urge incontinence occurs when a person senses the urge to void but is unable to inhibit leakage long enough to reach the toilet. In most cases, inhibited bladder contractions contribute to the incontinence. In patients with advanced cancer, central nervous system involvement by primary brain tumors or metastatic lesions may cause urgency leading to incontinence. Also, bladder tumors or other cancers involving the bladder may cause local irritations, which often are manifested as ur-gency (Herwig 1980).

Overflow incontinence occurs when the bladder is unable to empty normally and becomes overly distended, leading to frequent urine loss. Lesions in the true pelvis involving the peripheral pelvic nerves can often cause overflow incontinence. Any factor that causes outflow ob-struction, such as direct invasion of the bladder by a cancer, can lead to uncontrolled loss of urine due to overflow. Also, the mechanical effects of fecal impaction often lead to overflowing incontinence (Wrenn 1989).

Many types of urinary incontinence fall into the mixed category, displaying various aspects of more than one of the major subtypes. Occasionally a urinary fistula, such as vesicovaginal, presents with in-continence in patients with extensive pelvic cancer. As a result of radi-cal pelvic surgery, spinal cord compression below T11, damage to the sacral plexus, or an episode of outlet obstruction, a hypotonic bladder may develop. Features include difficulty in starting micturition, an intermittent stream, incomplete emptying, stress incontinence, persis-tent dribbling incontinence, and repeated infections (Regnard and Mannix 1991).

The term *functional incontinence* is applied to those patients in whom the function of the lower urinary tract is intact but other factors such as immobility or severe cognitive impairment result in urinary incontinence. This category is highly applicable to chronically ill patients.

In occasional circumstances, urinary incontinence may be related to prior cancer therapy. For example, treatment with cyclophosphamide can cause bladder wall fibrosis, leading to pronounced contraction of the bladder and loss of compliance. Radiation therapy has a similar effect (Herwig 1980).

It is clear that urinary incontinence is caused by multiple, often interacting factors. It is important to identify the reversible conditions such as infection, delirium, and drugs.

As with other symptoms in the dying patient, a clinical evaluation for possible causes of urinary incontinence is of paramount importance. The patient should not be relegated to the discomfort of an indwelling catheter until correctable conditions have been thoroughly explored. A careful history and physical examination with special attention to the preillness voiding pattern often produce an accurate diagnosis. Simple laboratory measurements, including urinalysis, serum creatinine or blood urea nitrogen levels, urine cultures, and postvoid residual urine volume, may be clinically helpful.

MANAGEMENT

The management of urinary incontinence in terminally ill cancer patients generally includes the use of drugs and protective devices. Behavior therapy, while highly successful in areas such as nursing homes, has limited use in terminal care because of the time necessary to train patients in these techniques.

The pharmacologic therapies currently used in the management of urinary incontinence have not been studied in well-designed clinical trials. Nonetheless, it has been suggested that many agents are beneficial for patients with urge incontinence due to uninhibited contractions of the bladder outlet muscle. Since these drugs increase the bladder's capacity, they may precipitate the retention of urine. Bladder relaxants include the anticholinergics, direct smooth muscle relaxants, calcium channel blockers, and imipramine.

Alpha-adrenergic agonists act as stimulants on the bladder outlet. These drugs produce smooth muscle contraction at the bladder outlet and may improve stress incontinence.

Protective devices available include absorbent pads or garments, indwelling catheters, and external collection devices such as condom catheters. Absorbent pads or garments are convenient temporary devices but are not suitable for long-term use. For men, external collection devices may be useful but are associated with an increased incidence of urinary tract infection. Practical external collection devices for women are not generally available (Consensus Conference 1989). Chronic indwelling catheters, which are often necessary in the terminal setting, invariably lead to urinary tract and systemic infections. Herwig (1980) thought that self-catheterization, when possible, is more physiologic and is better tolerated by the patient. Also, intermittent catheterization is the treatment of choice for patients with a hypotonic bladder (Regnard and Mannix 1991).

Pressure Sores

Pressure sores or decubitus ulcers are a serious problem for the hospitalized or homebound bedridden patient. The prevalence of this problem ranges from 3 to 11 percent. The in-hospital mortality rate in patients with pressure sores is between 23 and 37 percent (Allman 1989). Complications include osteomyelitis and sepsis. Recently, Hanson et al. (1991) reported a 13 percent incidence of pressure sores among hospice patients, with more than half (62 percent) occurring within two weeks of patient death. Because dying patients are chronically bedridden, the occurrence of pressure sores adversely influences the quality of life and, thus, prevention of this problem is of utmost importance.

The term *decubitus ulcer* (derived from the Latin word *ducub*, meaning "lying down") is often used to describe this problem. However, this is a misnomer, since a large number of these sores develop while the patient is in a sitting position (Reuler and Cooney 1981). Therefore, the term *pressure sore* is more accurate and describes the underlying pathophysiology.

Causes

Although many factors contribute to the development of pressure sores, four have been identified as critical: pressure, shearing forces, friction, and moisture. Pressure is the essential element. In the skin, the normal internal capillary pressure is 32 mm Hg. When external pressures greater than this amount are applied, the skin capillaries as well as the lymphatics collapse, leading to significant disruption of blood and lymphatic flow. The net result of this heightened pressure is time dependent. A pressure of 70 mm Hg applied for more than two hours produces irreversible tissue damage; if the same pressure is applied repeatedly for five minutes alternating with five minutes of no pressure, few changes occur. External pressures are higher in areas where soft tissue overlies bony prominences. Therefore, the great majority of pressure sores are located in the lower part of the body, with the sacral and coccygeal areas, ischial tuberosities, and greater trochanter accounting for the majority of pressure sore sites.

Shearing forces are another causative factor in the development of sores. Clinically, these forces are working when the head of the bed is raised, causing the body to slide down, transmitting pressure to the sacrum and deep fascia. At the same time, the posterior sacral skin is fixed, because of friction with the bed, and shearing forces in the deep part of the superficial fascia lead to stretching and distortion of blood vessels, which causes thrombosis and undermining of the dermis.

Friction is the force generated when two surfaces in contact move across each other, as when a patient is dragged across the bedsheets. Friction removes the outer protective layer of skin, accelerating the onset of ulceration. The final critical factor is moisture, caused by fecal or urinary leakage or perspiration, increasing the risk of pressure sore formation fivefold (Reuler and Cooney 1981).

RISK FACTORS

Although pressure, shearing forces, friction, and moisture are the causes of pressure sores, other factors place a patient at risk for developing this problem. To define further those factors associated with the presence of a pressure sore among adult patients hospitalized at Johns Hopkins Hospital, Allman et al. (1986) studied one group of patients with pressure sores and another group of patients at risk. The group at risk were patients who had been or were expected to be confined to a bed or chair for at least one week. Among 634 adult patients, 30 (5 percent) had a pressure sore and 78 (12 percent) were at risk. Furthermore, cancer was the only variable noted significantly more often among patients at risk. Comparing the patients with sores to the patients at risk, the authors found that fecal incontinence, diarrhea, fractures, use of urinary catheters, decreased weight, dementia, and hypoalbuminemia were associated with having a pressure sore. In addition, the authors reported that the presence of hypoalbuminemia, fecal incontinence, and fractures helped to identify bedridden patients at greater risk for developing pressure sores.

In a more didactic and less scientific fashion, Duffield (1989) listed both intrinsic and extrinsic factors predisposing to the development of pressure sores. Intrinsic factors are old age, debility, immobility, sedation or impaired consciousness, loss of sensory or motor function, spasticity, emaciation or obesity, malnutrition (especially vitamin C and protein), anemia, fever, edema, peripheral vascular disease, urinary and fecal incontinence, dehydration, and electrolyte imbalance. Extrinsic factors include loss of the skin's natural acidity (soap, laundry, or bed linen) or bacteria (disinfectants); repeated injections at vulnerable sites; poor nursing technique (e.g., body contact with impervious plastic); and systemic corticosteroids, nonsteroidal anti-inflammatory drugs, and chemotherapy and radiation therapy (table 2.8).

PREVENTION

The old adage "an ounce of prevention is worth a pound of cure" certainly applies to the area of pressure sores. In 1987, Colburn suggested a preventive strategy for pressure sores in hospice patients, which includes

- relieving pressure, especially over all bony prominences;
- maintaining the skin's integrity by keeping the skin clean and as free as possible from contamination with urine and feces;
- improving nutritional status by correcting nutritional deficiencies and promoting adequate hydration;
- promoting patient movement by providing active and passive motion as well as frequent turning;
- educating the patient and family regarding the need for a prevention program and the family's role.

Clearly the dictum "where there is no pressure, there is no sore" must not be forgotten (Reuler and Cooney 1981).

MANAGEMENT

Once a pressure sore occurs, management varies widely, often depending on local preference. Multiple topical therapies, various anti-pressure devices, and specialized beds have been advocated on the basis of uncontrolled, observational studies. In a randomized clinical trial, Allman et al. (1987) compared the use of air-fluidized beds to conventional therapy for pressure sores in hospitalized patients. Air-fluidized beds contain ceramic beads covered by a closely woven polyester sheet. Pressurized, warm air is forced up through the beads, which take on the characteristics of a fluid. Patients float on the bed without pressure on bony prominences. Other benefits include a dry environment, a freely movable surface, and a bacteriostatic bead system. Patients allocated to conventional therapy were to be repositioned at least every two hours, permitted to use heel and elbow protectors, and placed on a vinyl alternating air mattress covered by a 19-mm-thick foam pad. The

Table 2.8 The Risk Factors
for Developing Pressure Sores

Immobility
Elderly age
Nutritional deficiency, especially vitamin C
Age-related skin changes
Urinary and fecal incontinence
Diarrhea
Hypoalbuminemia
Pressure of a fracture
Dementia
Sedation or impaired consciousness
Loss of sensory or motor function
Emaciation or obesity
Anemia
Fever
Edema
Peripheral vascular disease
Dehydration
Electrolyte imbalance
Repeat injections at vulnerable sites
Poor nursing techniques
Drugs
Chemotherapy and radiation therapy
Pain

Sources: Allman (1989); Duffield (1989); Ryan
(1989).

air mattress was placed on top of the regular hospital bed. Patients
assigned to air-fluidized beds were to be repositioned every four hours.
In both groups, physicians were allowed to order a plastic surgery
consult, topical treatment with saline or povidone-iodine, enzymatic
debridement with a combination preparation of fibrinolysin and de-
oxyribonuclease, sterile gauze dressings, and whirlpool therapy as
needed. Thirty-one patients were randomized to the air-fluidized bed,
and 34 patients received conventional care. Overall, the results showed
that the air-fluidized beds are more effective than conventional therapy, especially for large sores. The use of the air-fluidized bed was associated with a significant reduction from the baseline in both the intensity
of the pain and the level of discomfort. In addition, the authors
stressed the need to determine the effectiveness of air-fluidized beds in
long-term care settings.

    More recently, Clarke et al. (1990) reported an unusual complica-
tion with the use of air-fluidized beds, namely, concealed bleeding.
They described two cases in which blood drained rapidly into the

chamber of an air-fluidized bed. This hemorrhaging was not obvious, since no signs of blood were detected on the patient's dressing or bed surface. To monitor for occult blood loss with air-fluidized beds, they recommended the use of a latex sheet.

PROGNOSIS

It is very difficult to determine the prognosis for the healing of pressure sores. As a general rule, patients in the last few weeks of life who are deteriorating rapidly (deterioration noticed daily) are unlikely to show healing of anything but the most minor skin damage, and even wound cleansing may be incomplete. Slower deterioration (weekly) may allow some partial healing of shallow ulcers (<0.5 cm) if nutrition is adequate. Slow deterioration (monthly) may allow time to clean and heal deep ulcers (>0.5 cm) (Bale and Regnard 1989).

Summary

Nausea and vomiting are problems encountered frequently in dying patients. Indeed, one study (Reuben and Mor 1986b) found that 62 percent of patients with terminal cancer experienced nausea and vomiting at some time during their last two months of life. In addition, these investigators reported that only one-third of the nauseated patients had received an antiemetic prescription. The implication of this study is clear: physicians must better appreciate the influence of this symptom on the quality of life of dying patients and must manage it more aggressively. If a correctable cause, such as hypercalcemia, is identified, then it should be treated appropriately. If an uncorrectable cause, such as metastatic liver disease, is found, then every attempt must be made to control this problem using antiemetic drugs and/or nonpharmacologic interventions.

About one-half of patients with advanced cancer (Curtis, Krech, and Walsh 1991) and other disease experience anorexia that results in cachexia. Corticosteroids have been used widely for years to manage this anorexia-cachexia syndrome, but there is no sound, scientific support for this practice. Multiple studies have shown that corticosteroids can improve appetite and the patient's sense of overall well-being; however, no study reported weight gain. In addition, these drugs are not without side effects, which may only compound existing problems, such as weakness and confusion.

Megestrol acetate offers new promise for the management of anorexia and cachexia in patients with cancer and AIDS. Its exact mechanism of action is unknown, but it seems to be an appetite stimulant, and weight gain is due not to the accumulation of excess fluid but rather to increases in fat and body cell mass. The optimal dosage of megestrol acetate to stimulate appetite is in the range of 160 to 800 mg/day. However, treatment with megestrol acetate is not inexpensive: an 800-mg dose costs $15 to $20.

Nutrition and hydration are two very emotion-laded problems associated with the management of dying patients. With advanced disease, the patient's taste perception is negatively altered, especially in regard to meat and sweets. The goal of nutritional therapy at this point is to improve the quality and value of life. The patient is allowed to eat whenever and whatever she or he desires. To avoid conflict, the physician should reassure the family that dying patients want only enough food and water to keep them comfortable.

The issue of hydration is less clear-cut than that of nutrition. One group, predominantly physicians, feels that parenteral hydration, be it by the intravenous or the subcutaneous route, is the minimal standard of care for the dying patient. Nurses, on the other hand, generally espouse a different opinion, namely, that terminal hydration only enhances the body's secretions, which in turn causes a more painful death. The physician must recognize both sides of this argument. A patient's dying without all the trappings of parenteral fluids and without excessive pulmonary and gastrointestinal secretions is both more comfortable for the patient and more humane for the caregiver. To help the patient reach this end, the physician must spend time with the patient and family, discussing the hydration issue and reassuring them that the lack of parenteral fluids does not represent abandonment by the physician and that death with dehydration is painless.

Constipation is a common and often distressing problem in patients with advanced disease. Although the reason varies, a correctable cause, such as electrolyte imbalance, should be investigated and managed appropriately. The narcotic bowel syndrome is unusual; if it is diagnosed, a trial of a continuous subcutaneous infusion of metoclopramide should be started. The prevention of constipation is of utmost importance; to this end, high-fiber diets, ambulation, increased oral fluids, and the removal of barriers to defecation are encouraged. In addition, the routine administration of laxatives, such as senna or a mixture of senna and lactulose, on a schedule similar to that for opioid analgesics is effective.

The reported incidence of delirium in dying cancer patients ranges from 53 to 85 percent. As with other symptoms, a reversible cause should be sought and managed. Polypharmacy is often overlooked in this setting. If sedation is required, haloperidol is the preferred drug.

Despite the common misperception, serious depression is distinctly unusual in dying patients (5 to 15 percent). It can be treated with short-term supportive psychotherapy and psychopharmacologic drugs, such as the tricyclic antidepressants. Alprazolam, a second-generation anti-depressant, is useful in patients with anxiety associated with depressive symptoms. The great majority of dying patients do not wish for early death, and the true incidence of suicide in dying patients is unknown.

Dyspnea is the most common severe symptom before death. Modest doses of morphine (5 to 10 mg every four hours) effectively relieve this symptom, as can the use of a small bedside fan. Antibiotics and supplemental oxygen are rarely indicated. Occasionally, thoracocentesis provides transient relief of symptoms if a large pleural effusion is present. Excessive pulmonary secretions ("death rattle") are best managed with scopolamine (0.4 to 0.6 mg given every four to eight hours as required) along with morphine. Coughing, which occasionally accompanies shortness of breath, is best treated by escalating the dosage of opioids.

Urinary incontinence is an infrequent but troublesome problem in the care of dying patients. Just before death, this is managed by protective devices such as indwelling or condom catheters.

Approximately one in five dying patients develops pressure sores, and few of these heal. Simple measures, including good skin care, frequent positioning, and, if available, the use of air-fluidized beds, are effective comfort measures.

Chapter 3

Other Problems in Patients with Cancer

Malignant Intestinal Obstruction

Intestinal obstruction is a common clinical problem in patients with advanced cancer, particularly those with colorectal or ovarian cancer. When cancer recurs or extends in these patients in the form of either large or small bowel obstruction, medical management can be difficult because of the associated psychosocial issues. On one hand, the clinical picture often is characterized by a patient unable to eat and malnourished, with intermittent abdominal discomfort and pain, who has received extensive prior cancer treatment including surgery, radiation therapy, and chemotherapy. In view of these factors, the patient presents a poor risk for surgical intervention. On the other hand, the patient's family becomes increasingly frustrated at watching their loved one "waste away" because of an inability to sustain any significant nutrition. This, in turn, leads to intense pressure on the physician to "do something." With few exceptions, clinical situations like this one sharply focus on the question of the quality of life.

Causes

The exact incidence of intestinal obstruction in hospice patients is not known, but investigators from St. Christopher's Hospice in London estimated that 3 percent of all of their patients had intestinal obstruction (Baines, Oliver, and Carter 1985). This escalated to 10 percent in patients with colorectal carcinoma. This obstruction is frequently related to extrinsic pressure from extramural masses rather than tumor recurrence within the bowel lumen. These extramural masses usually arise from serosal metastases or implants on the small bowel or may be due to metastatic involvement of the omentum, peritoneum, or other abdominal structures. The result is that these extramural metastases adhere to several loops of bowel, which accounts for the clinical observation that multiple sites of obstruction are common in these patients. However, nonmalignant causes of obstruction can occur. Osteen et al. (1980) retrospectively reviewed 66 cases in which the patient developed intestinal obstruction after treatment for cancer. In 32 percent of these patients, a benign cause of intestinal obstruction was found, such as adhesions, internal hernias, or radiation enteritis. In the 62 percent where obstruction was due to malignant neoplasm, the following risk factors were identified: a prior diagnosis of colorectal carcinoma, the presence of known metastatic disease, advanced stage of the primary tumor at diagnosis, and a short interval since the initial treatment of the cancer.

Advanced ovarian carcinoma ranks second in tumor sites causing intestinal obstruction. Krebs and Goplerud (1983) studied bowel obstruction in advanced ovarian carcinoma in 98 patients. They devised a risk score for these patients and identified the following significant negative prognostic factors: age greater than 65 years, poor nutrition, liver involvement or distant metastases, severe ascites, failed combination drug therapy, and previous radiation therapy to the whole abdomen. Although the colorectum and ovary are the most common primary sites, other areas, including gastric organs, pancreas, urinary tract, cervix, endometrium, skin, peritoneum, breast, and lung, have been reported (Aranha, Folk, and Greenlee 1981; Baines, Oliver, and Carter 1985; Osteen et al. 1980; Turnbull, Guerra, and Starnes 1989).

Significant insight into the problem of malignant intestinal obstruction, including management, was provided by Baines, Oliver, and Carter (1985). They studied 40 patients with intestinal obstruction treated at St. Christopher's Hospice in London. The patients were 26 to 94 years old, with a mean age of 59. Thirty-eight were managed without surgery; their symptoms included nausea and vomiting (100 percent); abdominal pain caused by hepatomegaly, tumor masses, or distension (92 percent); intestinal colic or crampy abdominal pain (76 percent); diarrhea (34 percent); and constipation (13 percent). This study highlights the spectrum of clinical symptoms associated with intestinal obstruction. In addition, symptoms such as crampy abdominal pain and distension may be intermittent because the obstruction may be incomplete at initial presentation.

MANAGEMENT

The initial management of the patient with bowel obstruction is surgical evaluation. There are few patients with a single obstructing lesion or in whom previous operative findings do not preclude surgery. For the majority of cases surgical intervention is not feasible because of the presence of multiple sites of obstruction and the overall poor clinical condition of the patient. At this point, general medical management consists of the insertion of a nasogastric tube for suction and intravenous fluids to maintain electrolyte and fluid balance. Using this approach, Osteen et al. (1980) reported a 23 percent spontaneous resolution rate. This resolution occurred quickly, and there seemed to be little benefit in extending the nasogastric suction beyond three days. Unfortunately, this approach provided only a temporary solution, since 41 percent eventually required surgical decompression.

Of the 40 patients managed in St. Christopher's Hospice (Baines, Oliver, and Carter 1985), 92 percent had undergone surgery, predominantly a bypass procedure, at least once. In only 2 of these patients was further surgical intervention possible to relieve the obstructive symptoms. The remaining 38 were managed without surgery and without the discomfort of prolonged nasogastric suction and intravenous fluids.

The authors evaluated the response to their treatment regimens based on the severity of symptoms before treatment, the dosage of medication necessary for symptom control, and the frequency of medication needed to maintain control. Smooth muscle-relaxant drugs, such as loperamide, scopolamine, and atropine, completely controlled crampy abdominal pain in 68 percent of the patients.

In well over half of the patients, scopolamine or atropine was given by subcutaneous continuous infusion. In patients with abdominal pain related to hepatomegaly, tumor masses, or distension, 89 percent were rendered pain-free with varying regimens of morphine, oxycodone, and diamorphine (not available in the United States). Again, subcutaneous continuous infusions, especially with diamorphine, were used. Nausea and vomiting, however, were more difficult to control; in only 13 percent of the patients were these symptoms completely controlled.

The most effective antiemetic drugs were phenothiazines (prochlorperazine, chlorpromazine) and butyrophenones (haloperidol). The subcutaneous continuous infusion route was also used with haloperidol. Patients were encouraged to eat and drink liberally, and dehydration was not a problem. Diarrhea was controlled in 56 percent with loperamide and codeine. Constipation occurred in few patients, and it was treated with stool softener in those patients in whom a single rectal or colonic obstruction was suspected.

Not surprisingly, the survival time for the 38 patients treated without surgery was short—a mean of 3.7 months. This, however, is similar to other reported survival times (Aranha, Folk, and Greenlee 1981; Krebs and Goplerud 1983; Osteen et al. 1980). For example, Osteen et al. (1980) reported a median survival of 3.0 months after operation for

32 patients found to have obstructions by recurrent cancer. In the group of 20 patients with a nonmalignant cause of obstruction, 9 (45 percent) died of recurrent cancer, with a median survival time of 5.5 months after surgery.

A more recent study (Ventafridda, Ripamonti, Caraceni, et al. 1990) from the Pain Therapy and Palliative Care Division of the National Cancer Institute of Milan also demonstrated the effectiveness of this type of conservative management. Twenty-two inoperable symptomatic patients with malignant intestinal obstruction were managed with continuous subcutaneous or intravenous infusions of morphine, haloperidol, and scopolamine. Morphine, for pain, was started with an initial dose of 0.5 mg/kg, and the final range was 20 to 80 mg/day. Scopolamine, for crampy pain and hypersecretions, was instituted at a dose of 1 mg/kg, and the final range was 40 to 380 mg/day. Haloperidol was given for nausea and vomiting at a beginning dose of 0.05 mg/kg, and the final range was 2 to 15 mg/day. All drugs were given via an infusion pump. The mean age of the patients was 58 years, with a range of 40 to 80 years. The treatment lasted 2 to 50 days, with a mean of 13.4 days. Seventeen patients were treated at home, and 5 were treated in the hospital. In all cases, the continuous infusions were continued until death. Because of this approach, a nasogastric tube with suction was avoided in 19 of the 22 patients. In the remaining 3 patients with upper intestinal obstruction due to gastric, pancreatic, and hepatic cancers, it was necessary to insert a nasogastric tube because therapy with antiemetic drugs was ineffective. Intravenous fluids were administered to only 1 patient to relieve thirst. In the 21 other patients, thirst and dry mouth were managed by oral fluids, ice cubes, pieces of pineapple, or chewing gum. The investigators noted that the use of intravenous fluids raises the volume of gastrointestinal secretions and therefore increases vomiting. An analysis of the patient's self-descriptive records showed that, after two days of treatment, the pain score decreased by more than 80 percent from the initial value. Based on their experience, the authors concluded that, in terminal cancer patients, pain and vomiting from inoperable intestinal obstruction, excepting obstruction of the upper bowel, can be controlled with continuous parenteral infusions of analgesic and antiemetic drugs, in the hospital and at home, without recourse to the placement of a nasogastric tube or to intravenous hydration.

Problems with hydration seem to be related to the level of intestinal obstruction. Distal bowel obstruction (rectum, colon, and ileum) still provides sufficient mucosal surface area for fluid absorption to prevent symptomatic dehydration. More proximal bowel obstructions may cause mild symptoms such as a dry mouth, which can be treated by ice chips, oral fluids, and the like. Obstructions proximal to the midjejunum may require parenteral fluids to treat symptomatic dehydration, especially thirst. The majority of patients, however, do not require intravenous hydration. Obstructions in the duodenum or proximal jejunum cause gastric retention, with associated epigastric discomfort and large-volume vomiting. If this obstruction is partial and motility is impaired, the patient may be helped with metoclopramide. If obstruction is complete, however, nasogastric suction is occasionally required. As the patient's condition deteriorates, dehydration results in reduced vomiting, decreases pulmonary secretions, and lessens urinary incontinence. Dehydration is normal at the end of life (Regnard 1988).

Malignant Dysphagia

Dysphagia, or difficulty in swallowing, is a problem not infrequently encountered in dying patients. Sykes, Carter, and Baines (1988) described this symptom as a presenting complaint in 11.7 percent of the terminally ill patients they studied. The clinical consequences of dysphagia are malnutrition and dehydration, which often lead to conflict regarding management.

There are many possible causes for the symptom dysphagia, since the act of swallowing involves not only the gastrointestinal tract from the oropharynx to the lower esophagus but also brainstem control of this function. As a practical matter, dysphagia in the cancer patient is generally related to primary tumors in the head and neck, esophagus, and upper stomach, in addition to tumors that metastasize to lymph nodes in the mediastinum, causing external compression.

CAUSES

Sykes, Carter, and Baines (1988), from St. Christopher's Hospice and the Royal Marsden Hospital, retrospectively reviewed their experience with dysphagia in patients with terminal malignant disease. This symptom was identified in 92 of 797 consecutive patients admitted over a 15-month period. The severity of dysphagia was assessed according to the consistency of food that caused symptoms from firm solids to liquids. The perceived level of obstruction, the presence and location of any associated pain, and symptoms of oral dryness or soreness were also noted. Excluding the 42 patients who died within one week, 33 patients had objective evidence of dysphagia on assessment, whereas the remaining 17 had no clear-cut evidence of dysphagia on assessment. The majority of patients in this latter group had tumors remote from the upper gastrointestinal tract and presented with significantly less severe dysphagia than did the 33 patients with clinical confirmation of this symptom. The esophagus was the leading primary site (30 percent) in patients with clinical evidence of dysphagia, followed by stomach (15 percent), oropharynx (12 percent), non-Hodgkin lymphoma (10 percent), tongue (6 percent), and miscellaneous sites (15 percent). More than half of the patients were able to describe a roughly consistent region, either above or below the clavicles, where food or liquids seemed to stick. In addition, one-third of the patients complained of pain or discomfort in the same area. Most patients had difficulty swallowing soft solids and liquids of varying consistencies. Twenty-one of these 33 patients were examined by limited symptom-directed autopsy. Local obstruction in the upper gastrointestinal tract by primary, metastatic, or multifocal tumor was found in 81 percent. Multiple obstructions were present in four patients. Of the patients who had identified the level of the obstruction (i.e., above or below the clavicles), their descriptions were confirmed 92 percent of the time. The survival of these dysphagic patients did not differ significantly from the hospice average.

Although Sykes, Carter, and Baines (1988) demonstrated that almost all patients in their study with objective evidence of dysphagia after careful assessment had local obstructive disease due to tumor, there are causes for this symptom in addition to tumor compression. It is generally assumed that infection of the oral cavity with the fungus *Candida albicans* can cause dysphagia as well as other oral symptoms; however, Finlay (1986) questioned this relationship. Mouth swabs were taken at weekly intervals in 140 consecutive patients in the Strathcarron Hospice in England. Patients were queried regarding the presence or absence of a wide variety of oral symptoms. Dysphagia was reported in 21 percent of patients with positive *Candida* cultures and in 32 percent of patients for whom the culture was negative for *Candida*. This difference was not statistically significant. Also, no correlation was shown between *Candida* and other mouth symptoms except between white lesions of the mouth and positive *Candida* cultures. Finlay concluded that the results of this study do not confirm that oral *Candida* is associated with symptoms or signs in the mouth, although oral candidiasis is common among terminally ill patients. Oral *Candida* and symptoms were not affected by antifungal treatment with nystatin. The author surmised that infection with *C. albicans* may be the result rather than the cause of mouth problems, indicating that general oral hygiene is more important than is antifungal therapy.

In 1982, Carter, Pittam, and Tanner studied, both clinically and pathologically, a group of 17 terminally ill patients with advanced squamous cell carcinoma of the head and neck. More than half of these patients had combined clinical and pathologic evidence of perineural spread, and the incidence of nerve involvement detected morphologically was high (88 percent). Clinically, sensory changes predominated, with multiple nerve involvement occurring in one-third of the patients. The most important conclusion to emerge from this study was the identification of an apparently new dysphagia syndrome in patients with advanced carcinoma of the oropharynx. The clinical picture was one of complete or nearly complete mechanical obstruction, but little or no direct block was found at autopsy. The signs and symptoms were due to perineural invasion into the ipsilateral vagal trunk, variable involvement of the sympathetic chain, splinting of the pharynx by local fibrosis, and tumor in the soft tissue of the neck. The resultant effect was neuromuscular incoordination producing dysphagia. As stressed by the authors, the recognition of this syndrome is important because short-term palliation was achieved with dexamethasone, 8 mg daily.

MANAGEMENT

In the study by Sykes, Carter, and Baines (1988), all of the 33 patients with clinical evidence of organic dysphagia were treated conservatively. This management included

- dietary intervention to ensure a diet of the right consistency for each patient;
- strict maintenance of oral hygiene;
- pain control, by standard treatments such as morphine and antiemetic drugs as required;
- the use of dexamethasone, generally 4 to 12 mg daily, if the tumor was likely to respond or when an external obstruction from nodal metastases was present; and
- the occasional use of palliative radiation therapy.

The response to treatment was assessed for each patient. Overall, 58 percent of the patients showed a response to treatment, from complete resolution to improved intake of food of the same consistency. The most refractory dysphagia occurred in patients with combined primary and metastatic tumor. Only 3 of the 33 patients were thought to have died other than completely peacefully. Nasogastric intubation, parenteral feeding, and feeding gastrostomy were not utilized in this study. Although these techniques ensure adequate caloric intake, two of them are restrictive and all do not prevent the aspiration of saliva. Rather than adding worthwhile life at this stage of the disease, they may prolong an uncomfortable death.

Two techniques clinically relevant to the treatment of malignant dysphagia are intracavitary irradiation and endoscopic laser palliation. Forty patients with advanced carcinoma of the esophagus and gastric cardia received palliative therapy by intracavitary irradiation. As reported by Rowland and Pagliero (1985), 65 percent experienced relief of dysphagia. In a study from the Mayo Clinic, Ahlquist et al. (1987) were able to improve swallowing in approximately 80 percent of the 25 patients with advanced esophageal cancer treated with endoscopic laser therapy. A single laser treatment provided adequate palliation in more than half of the patients until the time of death. Furthermore, no laser-related mortality or major morbidity occurred.

Barr and Krasner (1991) reported their experience with endoscopic laser therapy in 40 patients with obstructing gastric and esophageal cancer causing dysphagia. The patients' swallowing ability significantly improved with laser therapy, and 58 percent of the patients died at home. The mean survival was 16 weeks.

Neuromuscular Dysfunction

Weakness, defined as a deficiency in strength or power, is a common symptom in terminal illness and is present in the vast majority of patients with advanced cancer. As noted by Lichter (1990), weakness in terminal illness may be related to neuromuscular disorders from a wide variety of causes (table 3.1). Also, other forms of neuromuscular dysfunction are occasionally encountered in patients with advanced cancer.

Causes

Several well-known (paraneoplastic) syndromes demonstrate the remote effects of cancer on neuromuscular function (Bunn and Ridgway 1989). Patients with either dermatomyositis or polymyositis have five to seven times the incidence of malignant neoplasms compared to the general population. Clinically, this syndrome is characterized by a gradually progressive muscular weakness occurring over a period of weeks to months. The weakness eventually stabilizes, is usually not disabling, and usually involves the proximal muscles. In the majority of cases, the myopathy and cancer present within one year of each other. The myasthenic syndrome (Eaton-Lambert) is another classic example of a cancer, most often small cell carcinoma of the lung, producing a

Table 3.1   The Neuromuscular Causes of Weakness
in Terminal Illness

Related to the Cancer	Unrelated to the Cancer
Nervous system damage by tumor to:	Transient ischemic attacks
Brain	Motor neuron disease
Spinal cord	Myasthenia gravis
Peripheral nerves	Parkinsonism
Carcinomatous neuropathy	Peripheral neuropathies due to:
Myopathy	Diabetes mellitus
	Nutritional disorders
	Alcoholism
	Systemic diseases

Source: Lichter (1990).

remote or paraneoplastic effect on the neuromuscular system. This myasthenic syndrome is characterized by muscle weakness and fatigue, which are most pronounced in the pelvic girdle and thigh. Other common features include dryness of the mouth, dysphagia, dysarthria, and peripheral paresthesia. Successful treatment of the underlying small cell lung cancer can produce improvement in the muscular symptoms. Finally, the association of myasthenia gravis and thymoma is well established. Patients with myasthenia gravis present with muscular weakness, especially in the ocular and cranial muscles. There is a tendency for fluctuation and partial reversibility by cholinergic drugs. A number of tumors, including lymphomas and those of the pancreas, breast, prostate, ovary, thyroid, cervix, kidney, rectum, and palate, have been described in association with myasthenia gravis, but the incidence is the same as that expected in the normal population.

Bruera, Brenneis, Michaud, Jackson, et al. (1988), from the Cross Cancer Institute, Edmonton, Canada, prospectively studied 61 consecutive patients with advanced breast cancer to assess muscle electrophysiology. This group of patients was compared to 20 normal age- and sex-matched female controls. Nutritional status, lean body mass, voluntary and involuntary muscle electrophysiology tests of the adductor pollicis, and ultrasonographic measurement of the triceps brachialis, sternomastoid, and adductor pollicis muscles were determined in patients and controls. Patients with breast cancer were chosen because the incidence of malnutrition is significantly lower in this population than in patients with other cancers, such as lung or gastrointestinal. Malnutrition alone has been reported as a cause of abnormal muscle electrophysiology. The function of the adductor pollicis muscle of the hand was assessed because patients with advanced cancer still use the hand, as compared to muscles of the upper or lower limbs, which tend to atrophy with disuse. In addition, tumor mass and Karnofsky performance status were determined in the patient group. The nutritional status and the lean body mass did not differ significantly between patients and controls. Also, ultrasound studies of the three muscle groups failed to reveal any difference between patients and controls. There was, however, a difference in the muscle electrophysiology tests, with the cancer patients demonstrating abnormalities. These abnormalities were not correlated with tumor mass, performance status, the site of the primary breast cancer (right versus left), the use of chemotherapy known to cause nerve damage (vincristine), or the number of chemotherapy courses.

The authors concluded that they were unable to determine by their study the reason for the abnormal muscle electrophysiology in the patients with advanced breast cancer. They emphasized the importance of more research in this area as well as the major role that this muscular dysfunction may play in producing clinical symptoms such as weakness.

Muscle Cramps

Muscle cramps generally have been regarded as a nuisance but as benign, whatever the clinical setting. This perception has now been challenged by Steiner and Siegal (1989), who prospectively studied 50 cancer patients with new complaints of muscle cramps. Cramps were defined as localized, painful, involuntary skeletal muscle contractions of sudden onset. All patients were evaluated with a detailed neurologic examination and extensive laboratory and radiologic studies. The 50 patients included 36 women and 14 men who ranged in age from 12 to 80 years. The majority of patients had solid tumors, with the breast as the most frequent site. Most patients suffered frequent attacks that commonly occurred in both the upper and the lower extremities. Nocturnal cramps were described by slightly more than half of the patients.

In 41 patients (82 percent), a specific neural, muscular, or biochemical abnormality was identified as the most likely cause of muscle cramps. Most abnormalities were related to the peripheral nervous system. Muscle disease and biochemical abnormalities infrequently caused cramps. The use of amitriptyline resulted in a peripheral neuropathy in one case. In 9 patients (18 percent), no identifiable pathologic condition could be established. In two-thirds of the patients, muscle cramps were the first symptom of a previously unrecognized pathologic process.

Muscle cramps in cancer patients should not be ignored and frequently highlight the presence of an identifiable neurologic disorder (Steiner and Siegal 1989). Furthermore, the use of simple clinical and laboratory measures often leads to a diagnosis in the majority of patients.

Malignant Ulceration

Although the occurrence of malignant ulceration in patients with advanced and uncontrolled cancer is not especially common (8 percent) (Hockley, Dunlop, and Davies 1988), it is very distressing to both the patient and the family. The disagreeable odor of these large, fungating tumors often deepens the patient's sense of helplessness, embarrassment, and social isolation.

CAUSES

Wood (1980) categorized the location of malignant ulceration by anatomic site, namely, head and neck, thorax, perineum, abdomen, and extremities. Head and neck lesions are frequently of squamous cell origin and are especially difficult to treat. Generally, these patients have been treated with surgery, radiation therapy, and chemotherapy before the disease recurs. Complications of large, fungating head and neck tumors include airway obstruction and the invasion of major blood vessels with the possibility of erosion and fatal hemorrhage. A tracheostomy may be required to maintain an open airway. Lesions overlaying the carotid artery occasionally erode into the artery, with catastrophic and often fatal bleeding.

The major lesion in the thorax is female breast cancer and, less often, large sarcomas that may encompass the abdominal region as well. Perineal ulcerating wounds are frequently seen after the recurrence of a gynecologic cancer. The formation of a fistula is often an associated problem. Rectovaginal, rectovesical, or rectoperineal fistulas are best treated by permanently diverting the fecal stream, as with an end-colostomy. On the other hand, vesicovaginal or vesicoperineal fistulas are difficult to manage. Procedures to divert urine are usually not practical in these patients because of their short survival. Another complication of perineal ulceration is the presence of a constant bloody ooze.

Abdominal cancers can grow out of stomas and drain sites, causing obstruction, bleeding, and necrosis with malodorous sequelae. A related problem is that of subcutaneous and fascial infections adjacent to ulcerating tumors on the abdominal wall. Finally, large fungating lesions may involve the extremities and, in some instances, require palliative amputation.

MANAGEMENT

The smell of malignant ulceration is due to the presence of anaerobic organisms. These organisms flourish in the accessible necrotic tissues of fungating tumors, and the malodorous volatile fatty acids are released as a metabolic end-product. These fatty acids are responsible for the offensive and penetrating smell (Editorial, Smelly tumours, 1990). Brusis and Luckhaupt (1989) studied 31 patients with extensive tumors of the head and neck that emitted a putrid odor. Bacteriologic examinations were done either on smears of the ulcerating tumors or on samples of the tumors themselves. Distinct populations of anaerobes were always present. The most frequently demonstrated organism was *Bacteroides melaninogenicus*. This *Bacteroides* species, the authors thought, was responsible for the fetid odor.

Good local care is of utmost importance in managing patients with this problem. Keeping the area of the fungating mass dry and clean often prevents superimposed infections. Wood (1980) suggested cleansing with an inexpensive solution consisting of equal parts of hydrogen peroxide and normal saline. After twice-daily lavage, a small gauze packing soaked in 0.25 percent Dakin solution (sodium hypochlorite) overnight helps to lessen the smell. Daily charcoal dressing, which absorbs the volatile fatty acids, is sometimes sufficient to control the odor (Editorial, Smelly tumours, 1990; Ashford et al. 1984). Topical honey and icing sugar have also been suggested (Editorial, Smelly tumours, 1990). This preparation is thought to act by absorption and by the creation of a hyperosmolar environment that prevents bacterial growth. However, the sterility of honey is not assured, and neither agent is practical to use.

Another complication of malignant ulceration is a constant bloody drainage, especially with perineal lesions. Packing the wound with gauze or coagulation material such as absorbable gelatin sponge can sometimes slow this blood loss. In those instances where the mass is large and encompasses a whole region with hemorrhagic potential, major vessel ligation should be considered.

A unique palliative approach of radical surgical debridement for uncontrollable, recurrent pelvic tumors ulcerating through the perineum was described by Temple and Ketcham (1990). Seven patients, with a mean age of 61 years, were treated surgically with tumor resection including a portion of the sacrum to obtain all but the deep margins clear of tumor. Coverage was maintained with myocutaneous flaps. All patients had cancers that had failed to respond to treatment with chemotherapy and radiation. After the surgical debridement, all patients achieved significant pain relief. Three of the seven patients returned to work, and the remaining four led a relatively comfortable existence at home until death. The median survival of six patients after surgery was 11 months. At the time of the report, one patient was alive at 13 months.

The deodorizing effect of metronidazole was first described in 1980 and then confirmed in 1984. Ashford et al. (1984) performed a prospective double-blind, cross-over trial comparing metronidazole with placebo in nine patients with recurrent breast cancer. In all patients the smell was troublesome. Metronidazole was given for 14 days at a dosage of 200 mg three times daily in the treatment arm of the study. The smell was significantly less after metronidazole than after placebo, as was the difference in anaerobic isolates. According to the authors, the results clearly showed that metronidazole eliminated anaerobes and reduced the smell of fungating tumors. The net effect was an improvement in the quality of life of their patients with malodorous tumors.

In a similar vein, Brusis and Luckhaupt (1989) gave their patients with head and neck tumors either metronidazole or clindamycin to control the smell. Sixteen patients were treated with clindamycin (two 150-mg capsules four times daily), and 15 were treated with metronidazole (one 250-mg tablet five times daily). The odor disappeared more quickly after treatment with clindamycin than after treatment with metronidazole. The smell dissipated some 12 to 36 hours after the start of therapy.

Unfortunately, both clindamycin and metronidazole have drawbacks. Continuous therapy is necessary because the organisms soon regrow when the treatment is stopped. In addition, metronidazole can cause nausea, and long-term use is associated with neuropathy. The avoidance of alcohol that is necessary with metronidazole treatment may be difficult for some patients (Editorial, Smelly tumours, 1990).

To bypass these problems, some investigators have explored the use of topical metronidazole. Initial trials with dressings soaked in metronidazole injection preparation, although effective for bed sores and diabetic ulcers, were not totally successful in treating odorous tumors because the absorption was poor. Therefore, the metronidazole was incorporated in an 0.8 percent gel formation for use with daily dressings. A trial in 68 hospice patients with smelly tumors showed that it was totally effective in 50 percent, reasonably effective in another 46 percent, and ineffective in only 4 percent (Newman, Allwood, and Oakes 1989).

Summary

Malignant intestinal obstruction is an uncommon clinical problem (3 percent incidence in one series) (Baines, Oliver, and Carter 1985) but is difficult to manage. In inoperable cases, the continuous parenteral infusion of antiemetics, anticholinergics, and opioids provides a viable alternative to prolonged nasogastric suctioning and intravenous fluids. Thirst and dry mouth are relieved by oral fluids, ice chips, and the like. In cases where the obstruction is proximal (i.e., duodenum and proximal jejunum), nasogastric decompression may be necessary to reduce vomiting due to gastric retention. However, a trial of metoclopramide is appropriate if this obstruction is partial and motility is impaired.

Approximately 12 percent of dying cancer patients present with dysphagia, which is generally related to primary tumors in the head and neck, esophagus, or upper stomach and metastases to lymph nodes in the mediastinum. Although most patients with objective evidence of dysphagia have documented local obstruction, other causes for this symptom exist, including inadequate oral hygiene and the dysphagia syndrome due to poor neuromuscular coordination. Conservative treatment with diet, attention to oral hygiene, pain control, dexamethasone, and radiation therapy relieves dysphagia in about 60 percent of patients. Intracavitary irradiation and endoscopic laser therapy improve swallowing in more than half of patients.

Abnormal muscular function causing weakness seems to be unrelated to the patient's nutritional status, the size of the muscles, or the tumor mass. Presently, no specific treatment is available. Infrequently, paraneoplastic syndromes (for example, the Eaton-Lambert syndrome in patients with small cell lung carcinoma) produce muscular weakness as a remote effect of the cancer. The de novo appearance of muscular cramps is often associated with an underlying neurologic problem.

Although the occurrence of a large fungating tumor in a patient with advanced and uncontrolled cancer is not common (8 percent), it is very distressing to the patient and family. Good local care, especially keeping the area of the fungating mass dry and clean, is of utmost importance. Rarely, radical surgical debridement is necessary. Systemic drug therapy with metronidazole and clindamycin is effective in alleviating the odor of these tumors by reducing the offending anaerobic flora; however, it is impractical for long-term use. Topical metronidazole, on the other hand, is very effective in controlling the offensive smell.

Chapter 4

Other Problems in Patients
with Nonmalignant Diseases

Dementia

Progressive dementia of the Alzheimer type (DAT) is a neuro-degenerative disease with no cure. It affects approximately two million Americans and is probably the fourth leading cause of death among elderly people. Evidence suggests that the prevalence of DAT may be extremely high among very old people, nearing 50 percent in persons over 85 years of age. The length of survival with DAT is highly variable and may range from 2 to 16 years after the onset of symptoms (Walsh, Welch, and Larson 1990).

The hallmark of dementia is impairment of recent memory, but thought, judgment, perception, language, and functional abilities also deteriorate. Symptoms gradually worsen, and the clinical course is punctuated by acute intervening episodes. Behavioral symptoms include angry outbursts, violence, depression, suspicion, hallucinations, delusions, wandering, and other disturbing problems. The performance of simple tasks such as eating, dressing, and toileting eventually becomes impossible, and ultimately the patient needs long-term institutional care (Brechling and Kuhn 1989). The management of dementia consists of symptomatic treatment of behavioral problems, insomnia, seizures, and intercurrent illnesses.

In view of the similarities between Alzheimer disease and advanced cancer, it is not surprising that the hospice approach has been advocated for patients with dementia. Volicer et al. (1986) reported their experience in applying the hospice approach to 40 patients with advanced DAT in an intermediate care ward that constituted the inpatient component of the Alzheimer's Disease Research Program at the Bedford (Massachusetts) Division of the Boston Geriatric Research, Education, and Clinical Center.

The authors defined five levels of care depending on the optimality of treatment for each individual patient. The highest level (level 1) was aggressive care, including treatment of coexisting medical conditions, acute care transfer if necessary, and cardiopulmonary resuscitation if needed. The lowest level (level 5) was supportive care only. That care consisted of do-not-resuscitate orders, a decision not to transfer to an acute care unit, denial of work-up and antibiotic treatment of life-threatening infections (pneumonia, urinary tract infections), and the use of oral fluids only for hydration. Patients were assigned to a level of care after a meeting between the multidisciplinary team and family members. Of the 40 patients, none was assigned to level 1, whereas 19 patients (47.5 percent) were assigned to level 5. Although the environment and inpatient setting were different from conventional hospice care, the authors used similar philosophies and techniques to ensure maximal patient comfort. These included the maximization of quality of life by the use of recreational and occupational therapies, meticulous nursing care, attention to oral hygiene, the use of low doses of morphine if the patient was restless, the use of atropine to decrease pulmonary secretions, and the use of oxygen if the patient was dyspneic. With this approach, the authors believed that patients' suffering was minimized in the terminal stages of advanced DAT.

One of the clinically relevant aspects of Volicer et al.'s (1986) study was their identification and subsequent management of the infectious complications of advanced DAT. Of the 40 patients in the study, 13 died within the first year. An autopsy was performed in 11 cases, with the finding of pneumonia as the cause of death in 7 cases and sepsis resulting from urinary tract infections as the cause of death in 2 cases. Infection, therefore, was the most common cause of death in this advanced DAT population. The occurrence of pneumonia was often attributed to the aspiration of solids or liquids as a consequence of dysphagia, or difficulty in swallowing.

Sixty-two percent of the patients were not treated with antibiotics if they developed symptoms of pneumonia. The authors thought that the treatment of infections with antibiotics did not necessarily increase patients' comfort. The authors also did not favor empiric antibiotic therapy without a work-up and thought that the patients' comfort was maintained by the frequent use of analgesics and antipyretics. In addition, preliminary data indicated that the hospice approach did not significantly increase the mortality of patients with DAT.

Lynn (1986), in an accompanying editorial, found these clinical situations to be less clear. She suggested that the elderly demented person whose strength is being slowly drained by fever and cough should be given antibiotics and restored to his or her previous level of health.

In follow-up of their 1986 study, Fabiszewski, Volicer, and Volicer (1990) prospectively evaluated fever episodes in 104 institutionalized patients with DAT to determine the effect of antibiotic treatment on the outcome of fever. Fever was defined as an unanticipated rectal temperature elevation to 38.9°C or higher or a temperature of 37.7°C or higher that persisted for more than 24 hours. In patients assigned to the antibiotic group, each episode of fever was evaluated using a standardized protocol that consisted of the notation of subjective complaints, functional status assessment, physical examination, and a battery of radiologic and laboratory tests. During those episodes where the source of the fever was clinically apparent, broad-spectrum antibiotic coverage was started on the completion of the diagnostic protocol. In cases where no source of infection was obvious, the patient was monitored and treated with antipyretics and no antibiotics until the culture results were available. For the patients in the palliative group, each episode of fever was evaluated identically to that of the antibiotic group with the deletion of the diagnostic tests. These patients were treated symptomatically with antipyretics, analgesics such as morphine when needed, and other therapeutic modalities, including oxygen, oral hydration, pulmonary toilet, and intensive hospice-like nursing care. During the 34-month observation period, 75 patients developed 172 episodes of fever and 29 patients had no fevers. Fever was present more often in patients with advanced disease. Patients with fever treated with antibiotics were compared to patients with fever treated with comfort care only. The incidence of fever was similar for both groups of patients. A survival analysis showed that, for the more severely affected patients, there was no survival difference between the antibiotic and the palliative group; however, among the less severely affected patients, survival was higher for the antibiotic-treated patients. These results, as interpreted by the investigators, indicate that fever is a common occurrence in institutionalized patients with Alzheimer disease and that palliative care is an appropriate treatment option, especially for the more severely impaired patients with DAT.

Motor Neuron Disease

Motor neuron disease is a heterogeneous group of disorders with varying signs and symptoms, all affecting in some manner the anterior horn cells. The most common subset of motor neuron disease in adults is amyotrophic lateral sclerosis (ALS), which affects not only the anterior horn cells but also the corticospinal tracts. The net effect of the ALS lesion is progressive wasting and weakness of those muscles that have lost their nerve supply, in addition to corticospinal tract signs of spasticity and pathologic reflexes in the absence of sensory findings. In most cases of ALS, intellectual function remains intact. Variants of classic ALS include progressive muscular atrophy and progressive bulbar palsy. Atrophy of the spinal muscles presents a clinical picture of limb weakness and wasting with varying degrees of cranial nerve involvement. Progressive bulbar palsy is dominated by weakness and atrophy of cranial nerves of the lower motor neuron type (Williams and Windebank 1991).

The worldwide incidence of ALS is 0.4 to 1.8 per 100,000 people. The incidence of familial ALS is approximately 5 to 10 percent of all ALS. The male to female ratio is 1.0:1.6, and the age at onset is between 50 and 60 years (Mitsumoto, Hanson, and Chad 1988).

About one-third of patients with ALS notice the onset of disease because of fine motor impairment affecting activities like sewing or using tools. Another one-third present with leg weakness, while the remaining one-third complain of dysphagia or dysarthria due to involvement of the corticobulbar tract. Although the disease characteristically progresses to involve all muscle groups, involvement of the distal muscles is often more severe than involvement of the proximal muscles.

Weakness of bulbar musculature may cause varying degrees of dysarthria and/or dysphagia. The patient's speech may be difficult to interpret because of slowing, tongue weakness, or difficulty in articulation. The patient may have difficulty in initiating swallowing, and saliva may accumulate in the pharynx, leading to episodes of choking. Some patients may have a hyperactive cough reflex, whereas others may not be able to cough adequately, thus predisposing them to aspiration pneumonia.

The control of bladder, bowel, and autonomic function is generally unimpaired, even late in the disease. Another important feature of ALS is the surprising absence of pressure sores, even in patients bedridden for long periods (Mitsumoto, Hanson, and Chad 1988).

Because of the poor prognosis associated with ALS, it is important to confirm the clinical diagnosis by investigative procedures. Among the studies most essential is the electromyogram (EMG), which shows characteristic changes consistent with the diagnosis of ALS. Furthermore, the EMG may be useful in the early stages by establishing the widespread nature of the involvement. Occasionally, computed tomographic (CT) scanning of the spine and magnetic resonance imaging (MRI) are necessary to eliminate other diagnoses, such as degenerative disease of the spine with nerve compression, which can mimic ALS.

The clinical outlook for ALS is bleak, with an average survival of 3 years. One-half of the patients die in less than 3 years, with only 20 percent and 10 percent surviving more than 5 and 10 years, respectively. Younger patients with a longer duration before diagnosis and milder involvement at diagnosis have a better prognosis, whereas older patients with a shorter duration and more severe involvement at diagnosis have a poorer prognosis (Mitsumoto, Hanson, and Chad 1988).

Despite ongoing active clinical research, the cause of ALS remains obscure. Likewise, all therapeutic interventions have been uniformly ineffective. Thus, the major care for patients with ALS remains supportive, not curative.

In an attempt to understand better the problems of caring for patients with ALS and other motor neuron disease at St. Christopher's Hospice, Saunders, Walsh, and Smith (1981) retrospectively reviewed their experience with 100 patients. Forty men and 60 women were included in this survey. The median ages were 57 years for men and 64 years for women. The median stay in hospice for men was 80 days, with a wide range from 8 hours to four and one-half years. The women's stay in hospice was shorter, with a median of 32.5 days and a range of 11 hours to 157 weeks. Sixty percent of the patients had noted the onset of the disease between one and three years before admission. In the whole group, paralysis was generally widespread and communication was often difficult.

A wide range of symptoms was encountered in these patients. Common symptoms included constipation, dysarthria, dysphagia and choking attacks, dyspnea, insomnia, pain, salivation and secretions, and tiredness. Diarrhea was occasionally a problem, whereas pressure sores, hunger and thirst, and urinary problems were uncommon. The pharmacologic management of these troublesome clinical problems varied by symptoms, but often one drug was used in several different clinical situations. For example, opioids were employed in 84 percent of the patients for pain, dyspnea, misery, anxiety, insomnia, hunger, and thirst. A diazepam was given to 63 percent of the patients to control muscle fasciculations, spasticity, cramps, and anxiety. Finally, tricyclic antidepressants were used in 40 percent of the patients for depression, sadness, and insomnia.

As advocated by Saunders, Walsh, and Smith (1981), the skilled use of small doses of opioids can have a positive effect on the management of this disease. These drugs can be given as effective tranquilizers and hypnotics at an early stage of the disease. During their review, Saunders, Walsh, and Smith (1981) found that the maximal dose of parenteral diamorphine for most patients ranged between 2.5 and 5.0 mg.

A definition of pain was sought from 45 patients, with approximately half complaining of the combination of stiffness, aching, cramping, and burning discomfort. This symptom complex was often well controlled by the use of physiotherapy and also by the nonsteroidal anti-inflammatory drugs early and by opioid drugs later.

Parenteral diamorphine combined with chlorpromazine, diazepam, and/or anticholinergics was used for terminal distress of any kind. One or more injections were given in 75 percent of the patients. Of the 100 patients, 94 had died, only 1 in a choking attack.

Death was quick in the majority of cases. The most common clinical picture was of sudden rapid deterioration, frequently starting with an upper respiratory infection and followed by increasing exhaustion and dyspnea. Of the 10 autopsy examinations done, 6 showed widespread bronchial pneumonia.

Finally, the patients' moods ranged from depressed to anxious/frightened. Saunders, Walsh, and Smith (1981) thought that their emotional liability was a little greater than would be expected in a normal person with limited communication ability. The authors also stressed the importance of distinguishing sadness and frustration from a true depressive reaction. Of the 15 patients admitted to hospice on tricyclic antidepressants, only 4 were considered to be depressed on admission. On the other hand, 14 patients who were considered to be depressed were not receiving antidepressants. Some 40 percent of patients were treated with tricyclic antidepressives, not only for depression but also for sedation and the anticholinergic beneficial side effect. Only 14 percent of the patients were referred for psychiatric consultation. The investigators thought that dying of ALS was no more a psychiatric problem in itself than was dying of cancer.

In an updated review of the St. Christopher's experience, O'Brien, Kelly, and Saunders (1992) highlighted the response of symptom control to opioid treatment in 124 patients with motor neuron disease. Of the 57 percent of patients with pain, three-quarters obtained good pain control with opioids. Dyspnea, occurring in 47 percent of the patients, also responded favorably to the use of opioids in 81 percent of the cases. Insomnia, likewise, was well controlled with opioids in the great majority (82 percent) of patients with this problem (48 percent). The mean dose of opioid (oral morphine equivalent) was 30 mg/24 hours, and the mean duration of the treatment was 58 days. Many patients were noted to deteriorate suddenly, and in 58 percent of the cases death occurred within 24 hours of this deterioration. When dying, 106 patients (94 percent) were peaceful and relaxed; 101 patients (89 percent) received opioids during this dying period. No patient choked to death. In fact, the authors strenuously objected to the term *choking* and thought that it is both inappropriate and inaccurate in describing the cause of death in motor neuron disease. Furthermore, they advocated the abandonment of its use.

Acquired Immunodeficiency Syndrome

Since the initial description of AIDS in 1981, more than 179,000 cases of AIDS have been reported in the United States and more than half (63 percent) of these patients have died. The Centers for Disease Control (CDC) have estimated that there were approximately 750,000 HIV-infected individuals in the United States at the beginning of 1986 and that, as of late 1990, this number had increased to one million. At the current rate of progression of AIDS in HIV-infected individuals, it is estimated that there will be 390,000 to 480,000 cases of AIDS, with between 285,000 and 340,000 deaths, by the end of 1993 (Gold 1992).

Initially, AIDS was a disease of homosexual and bisexual men. In the United States, most cases still occur in this group. However, the number of cases in intravenous drug users is increasing, and this group and its sexual contacts now represent the largest group at risk. In 1990, heterosexual infection accounted for the most rapid increase in HIV infection. The incidence of new cases of AIDS acquired by blood transfusion and replacement of clotting factor has stabilized as a result of screening blood and blood products. The number of cases in infants born to HIV-infected women has increased, reflecting the spread of this infection to women, who now account for more than 10 percent of cases (Gold 1992).

Patients with AIDS have a wide variety of opportunistic infections and malignant neoplasms (Kaplan, Wofsy, and Volberding 1987). Of all the opportunistic infections, *Pneumocystis carinii* pneumonia is the most common. Patients generally present with fever, nonproductive cough, and exertional shortness of breath. Symptoms of cryptococcal meningitis include a high fever and headache. Toxoplasmosis is a common cause of central nervous system disease in patients with AIDS. Focal neurologic findings, seizures, fever, or a decreased level of consciousness is often found. *Cryptosporidium* is frequently associated with severe and chronic watery diarrhea, which can lead to dehydration and wasting. Both *Mycobacterium avium* and *Mycobacterium tuberculosis* infections are frequently seen in AIDS patients. Oropharyngitis due to candidal infection is the most common fungal infection encountered. It is present in the majority of patients with AIDS at some time during the course of the disease. Infections of herpes simplex virus are common and may be severe and persistent.

Cytomegalovirus (CMV) is a frequent cause of morbidity and mortality. CMV is often associated with pneumonitis, retinitis, cerebritis, or colitis.

Like the opportunistic infections, malignant neoplasms associated with AIDS (namely, Kaposi sarcoma and non-Hodgkin lymphoma) are difficult to treat. Since most patients with AIDS die of opportunistic infections rather than Kaposi sarcoma, treatment is aimed at reducing the morbidity of advanced Kaposi sarcoma, such as the bulky, painful skin or oropharyngeal lesions. Since neither antibiotic therapy for opportunistic infections nor chemotherapy and radiation therapy for malignant neoplasms are able to reverse the underlying immune defect in AIDS, new forms of treatment were developed specifically to affect this immunodeficiency state. One such treatment is the antiviral agent zidovudine (AZT). As reported preliminarily by Yarchoan and Broder (1987), the drug was given for up to 18 months in AIDS patients. The results showed an improvement in immunologic function, a reversal (at least partially) in neurologic dysfunction in some patients, and an improvement in certain other clinical AIDS-associated abnormalities. The average survival of 10 months that was originally reported in these patients has now been extended to approximately two years with the use of AZT (Redfield and Tramont 1989). AZT given to asymptomatic patients and to patients with AIDS-related complex (ARC) delays the onset of AIDS; however, the benefits of AZT therapy are not permanent, and AIDS will develop in most HIV-infected patients (Gold 1992).

Patients with advanced or terminal stages of AIDS share many of the same symptoms of patients dying of other diseases, such as cancer. Chronic infections and skin problems, however, are uniquely found in the dying AIDS patient. Moss (1991) retrospectively reviewed the first 100 consecutive admissions to a new palliative care unit for AIDS patients. The vast majority of the patients were men who had contracted the disease by homosexual contact or intravenous drug use. The ages ranged from 20 to 70 years, with 78 percent being between 30 and 49 years old. All of these patients had a number of coexisting diagnoses, usually three or four, and most of these were opportunistic infections for which active treatment, maintenance therapy, or prophylaxis was being given. For example, 68 percent of the patients had prior candidal infection and 64 percent of these were receiving active therapy or prophylaxis. More than half (59 percent) had had one or more previous episodes of *P. carinii* pneumonia, and 60 percent of these patients were taking prophylactic drugs. The 18 patients (22 percent) with a diagnosis of mycobacterial disease were taking several antituberculous drugs, and 22 patients (28 percent) had a diagnosis of cytomegalovirus retinitis. As a result of these coexisting problems, polypharmacy was inevitable. A total of 48 percent of the patients were taking 4 to 6 drugs, and 30 percent were taking 7 to 10 drugs. About one-third of the patients were receiving AZT and continued to do so until the very end. Pain was a frequently (84 percent) encountered symptom. Pain due to HIV-related demyelinating peripheral neuropathy was the most common (22 percent), followed by pain from pressure sores, visceral pain, total body pain, headache, joint pain, epigastric/retrosternal pain, muscle pain, and anorectal discomfort. Unlike the causes of pain in dying cancer patients, some sources of discomfort in AIDS patients were related to infections and drugs. For example, headaches were often associated with infections of the central nervous system, such as cryptococcal meningitis or cerebral toxoplasmosis. Retrosternal or epigastric pain usually was related to the presence of candidal esophagitis. Finally, myopathic pain correlated with the use of AZT, especially in high doses.

Other common symptoms noted by Moss (1991) were weight loss, anorexia, confusion, nausea and vomiting, depression, cough, diarrhea, constipation, dyspnea, and paralysis (table 4.1). Skin problems were extremely common (45 percent). About 20 percent of the patients had dry skin, which predisposed to bacterial skin infections. Tinea and other fungal infections were frequent. Fourteen percent of the patients had seborrheic dermatitis, which was often linked to fungal infections. Scabies infection was noted in 7 percent of the patients.

Psychiatric problems, such as anxiety and depression, are common

Table 4.1 Common Symptoms in 100
Patients with Advanced AIDS

Symptom	Frequency
Pain	84%
Weight loss	61%
Skin problems	45%
Anorexia	41%
Confusion	29%
Nausea and vomiting	21%
Depression	20%
Cough	19%
Diarrhea	18%
Constipation	18%
Dyspnea	11%
Paralysis	8%

Source: Moss (1991).

in AIDS patients but must be distinguished from AIDS-related dementia, which occurs in at least half of the patients before death. HIV has been shown to have direct effects on the central nervous system; nevertheless, most HIV-infected asymptomatic patients evidence no clinically significant mental changes. A few, however, show a subtle dementia characterized by apathy, social withdrawal, the avoidance of complex tasks, and mental slowing. As death approaches, more significant dementia develops, but at this point it is difficult to discern the degree to which the cognitive decline is due to the direct effects of HIV on the central nervous system, systemic illness, infection, tumor, or the effects of various medications (Jacobsberg and Perry 1992).

The control of pain and symptoms for terminally ill patients with AIDS is similar to that outlined for other diseases, such as cancer. Indeed, megestrol acetate has shown a salutary effect on appetite and weight gain in AIDS patients with anorexia and cachexia (Von Roenn, Murphy, and Weber 1990). No randomized clinical trial on the use of corticosteroids in patients with advanced AIDS has been reported, although Cole (1991) advocated their generalized use based on his personal experience.

Because of the known polypharmacy in AIDS patients, clinicians must consider stopping as many medications as possible to avoid undue toxicity and potential drug interactions. The treatment of candidiasis and prophylaxis against herpes simplex reactivation should be continued as long as possible, since the morbidity of these conditions is high and their progression does not cause a rapid demise. Although the treatment of mycobacterial disease occasionally produces a beneficial effect, it can be discontinued and fever and sweating can be controlled with antipyretic drugs.

It is also reasonable to stop parenteral therapy for cytomegalovirus retinitis, since more than half of patients do not develop progressive retinitis until three weeks after drug discontinuation or beyond. Since the benefit of AZT in advanced AIDS has not been established, this drug should also be stopped, with patient concurrence. Medications for pain and symptoms, such as acetaminophen, morphine, and nonsteroidal anti-inflammatories, compete with AZT for hepatic metabolism and can increase serum levels of AZT to potentially toxic heights. Finally, Cole (1991) did not personally observe reactivation or symptomatic progression of opportunistic infections after stopping treatment.

Anecdotal case reports have, on occasion, demonstrated that the transmission of HIV to a health care worker can result from various modes of exposure to HIV, such as contaminated hollow-bore needles with parenteral injury, cuts, mucosal splashes, or skin contact. Some cases of HIV transmission related to needlestick injury involved only limited blood infusion or a relatively superficial injury. Epidemiologic studies of occupational risks of transmission have shown that persons who have had parenteral exposure have the greatest risk (i.e., about 0.5 percent). The observed risk associated with known exposure via mucosal membrane and skin is close to zero (Weiss 1992).

Chronic Vegetative State

The care of terminally ill patients, especially those in a chronic vegetative state, can be very trying. Because of this, Carlson, Devich, and Frank (1988) developed a comprehensive support care team in a major teaching hospital to manage these patients. The team included a physician and a clinical nurse specialist who provided primary medical care, family support, and in-service guidance to the hospital staff about ethical issues. Nursing, pastoral care, social work, and other hospital services were incorporated into a multidisciplinary approach.

The goals of the comprehensive support care team were

- to provide a hospital service dedicated to consistent and humane care of the hopelessly ill patient and support of their families,
- to develop a treatment plan for each patient that reflected ethical decision making involving patient and proxy/family,
- to provide comprehensive but conservative care using a multidisciplinary approach,
- to facilitate access to institutional and community support services, and
- to promote learning about and discussion of ethical issues by the hospital staff.

During an 18-month period, 212 patients were accepted on the team's service. The mean age of the patients was 67 years, with a range of 17 to 100 years. The most common diagnosis was global central nervous system anoxia after cardiopulmonary arrest in 62 patients (29 percent). A variety of other neurologic disorders accounted for 79 patients (37 percent). Therefore, for 141 patients (67 percent) under the team's care, dysfunction of the central nervous system was a major clinical feature. Diagnoses in the remaining patients included cancer (16 percent), gastrointestinal (predominantly hepatic) failure (7 percent), renal failure (4 percent), pulmonary failure (2 percent), metabolic abnormalities (2 percent), cardiovascular problems (1 percent), and acquired immunodeficiency syndrome (1 percent). Most patients (78 percent) were receiving mechanical ventilation when accepted on the service. About one-third of these patients were weaned from assisted ventilation. An additional 17 percent were terminally weaned with discontinuation of ventilatory life support. The mean length of the hospital stay was 26 days for all patients, with a mean length of stay under the care of this team of 9 days. Only 6 patients (3 percent), all comatose, were discharged home; another 25 patients (12 percent) were transferred to an extended care facility. The remaining patients either died (82 percent) or were returned to their primary care service (3 percent). Survival rates were very similar when comparing before, early, and late management by the team in patients with global anoxic brain injury. However, there was a progressive decrease in the length of stay in the hospital corresponding to the full development of the team service. It was the authors' hope that this approach to the care of the terminally ill, especially those in coma, would serve as an alternative method of treatment in similar hospital settings.

Advanced Pulmonary Disease

Advanced pulmonary disease, usually due to chronic bronchitis or emphysema, is very similar to advanced cancer in that it is progressive, is incurable, and causes distressing symptoms, ultimately leading to death (Kinzel 1991). The treatment of the symptoms of patients with advanced pulmonary disease is the same as that previously described for other terminal diseases except in the management of hypoxia, infections, dyspnea, and panic attacks.

Hypoxia is present in the majority of symptomatic patients with advanced pulmonary disease. The hemoglobin oxygen saturation should be maintained above 90 percent, with supplemental oxygen to maintain the function of the cardiovascular and central nervous systems.

Recurrent pulmonary infections are common in advanced pulmonary disease and frequently are the cause of death. When death is not imminent, treating the pulmonary infection is essential in relieving dyspnea. Treatment is usually empiric. Broad-spectrum antibiotics should be started when shortness of breath worsens and is associated with a change in sputum or when other signs of infection are present.

Dyspnea is the cardinal symptom in patients with advanced pulmonary disease. It may be caused by hypoxia, congestive heart failure, tenacious secretions, minor infections, ischemic heart disease, pleural effusion, reflux esophagitis, or emotional distress. Because there is no uniformly effective method of alleviating dyspnea, the clinician should search for and appropriately manage any complicating medical conditions, such as congestive heart failure. Pulmonary function should be optimized by good pulmonary toilet, theophylline, inhaled or oral beta agonists, inhaled atropine derivatives, steroids, and low-flow oxygen. Theophylline can be given effectively orally with a once-daily preparation, usually given at bedtime. The blood levels of theophylline should be monitored periodically to minimize toxicity. Beta agonists, mainly albuterol or metaproteranol, are administered by a hand-held multi-dose inhaler, usually with a spacer device. Two inhalations four times daily is the standard dose; however, in very late stage patients who benefit from inhaled beta agonists, doses may be increased to three inhalations every four hours. Ipratropium (an atropine derivative) may also be helpful when used as two inhalations four times daily. Finally, morphine in dosages of 2.5 to 10 mg orally every four to six hours is useful in relieving dyspnea.

Panic is the most dramatic emotional symptom in patients with advanced pulmonary disease. It is associated with a rapid exacerbation of symptoms into a vicious cycle: panic causing increased bronchospasm, leading to increasing dyspnea, leading to further panic. Strong emotional support, along with an increase in the inhaled beta agonist, may relieve minor attacks. Treatment with 0.25 mg subcutaneous terbutaline or 3 to 5 mg subcutaneous morphine is more effective (Kinzel 1991).

Summary

Progressive dementia of the Alzheimer type has no cure. Like advanced cancer, it follows a relentless downhill clinical course punctuated by acute intervening episodes, predominantly infectious in nature. For severely impaired patients, the management of the symptoms of these episodes (generally pneumonia) with antipyretics, analgesics, and intensive nursing care produces the same outcome as does more aggressive treatment using diagnostic tests and antibiotics.

Likewise, there is no curative therapy for motor neuron diseases such as ALS; there is only supportive care. Common symptoms include dysarthria, dysphagia, choking attacks, dyspnea, constipation, insomnia, pain, salivation, excessive secretions, and tiredness. Small doses of opioids are extremely effective in managing not only pain but also other symptoms.

Patients with AIDS encounter many of the same problems as patients dying of other diseases. Chronic infections and skin disorders, however, are uniquely found in the patient dying of AIDS. Pain is the most frequent symptom and is often due to HIV-related demyelinating peripheral neuropathy. The control of pain and other symptoms in these patients is very similar to that outlined for other diseases, including the use of megestrol acetate for anorexia and cachexia. Avoid polypharmacy to prevent undue toxicity and drug interactions.

The use of a comprehensive support care team to manage the comatose patient in a chronic vegetative state is an enlightened approach to a most difficult problem.

The treatment of the symptoms of patients with advanced pulmonary disease differs from that of other terminal illnesses in the management of hypoxia, infections, dyspnea, and panic attacks. Use supplemental oxygen for hypoxia, and administer antibiotics for pulmonary infections. To lessen dyspnea, optimize pulmonary function by good pulmonary toilet and the use of theophylline, beta agonists, atropine derivatives, steroids, low-flow oxygen, and low doses of morphine. Manage panic attacks with strong emotional support, inhaled beta agonists, terbutaline, or small doses of morphine.

Chapter 5

Palliative Surgery

Although surgical intervention is infrequent in dying patients, palliative surgery plays an important role, much like chemotherapy and radiation therapy, in the management of these patients' symptoms. As noted by Forbes (1988), the overall goal of palliative surgery is to improve the patient's quality of life by appropriately reducing symptoms without undue surgical complication. To this end, Forbes reviewed the basic principles relevant to the surgical management of patients with advanced cancer (table 5.1).

- Patients with cancer undergoing surgery are primarily surgical patients. Therefore, it is important to address the physical and psychologic stresses generally associated with any surgical procedure.
- Surgery is directed at the consequences of the tumor. Morbidity in advanced cancer often results from the anatomic location of the tumor. For example, advanced head and neck cancers have the potential to erode the carotid artery, resulting in dramatic and explosive bleeding. Palliative surgery can prevent this event. Hence, surgical intervention in patients with advanced cancer should be aimed at the symptoms rather than at the overall malignant process.
- Integrate surgery into both specific treatment and supportive care programs. Surgery for palliation must be an integral part of the total management plan for the patient.
- Avoid unreasonably delaying palliative surgery. The patient's quality of life is best improved by quickly relieving the distressful symptoms and by avoiding the anxiety associated with the uncertainty of future management plans.
- Surgical problems may have a benign cause; obtain histologic findings where possible. The following examples of definitive palliative surgery illustrate the uncertain intent of surgery before the

Table 5.1   An Overview of Palliative Surgery

The role of surgery in palliation:
  Cancer patients are surgical patients first.
  Surgery is directed at the consequences of the tumor.
  Integrate surgery into both specific treatment and supportive care programs.
  Avoid unreasonable delay of palliative surgery.
  Surgical problems may have a benign cause; obtain histological findings where
    possible.
Principles of preoperative care:
  Consultations and explanations should be done.
  Preoperative planning for immediate and long-term care is important.
Principles of operating for advanced cancer:
  Incisional site must be determined.
  Each patient must undergo the procedure that is optimal for him or her.
Principles of postoperative care:
  Optimize recovery by avoiding complications.
  Early diagnosis and aggressive management of complications are important.

Source: Forbes (1988).

procedure. Patients with obstructive jaundice and known cancer may have liver metastases, extrahepatic biliary obstruction due to lymph node metastases, or a benign disease such as cholelithiasis. In this case, surgical exploration will establish the cause of jaundice and, if feasible, appropriate surgery can be performed. Intestinal obstruction may well be due to recurrent or progressive disease in patients with known ovarian or colorectal cancer. However, in one-third of the cases, the obstruction will be caused by a benign process such as adhesions, internal hernias, or radiation enteritis.

The Principles of Preoperative Care

- The burdens and benefits of the planned surgery must be carefully explained to the patient and family. Likewise, anticipated outcomes without surgical intervention should be fully discussed with the patient and family.
- Preoperative planning for immediate and long-term care is essential. The results of palliative surgery may depend largely on the adequacy of the preoperative preparation and assessment. Cancer patients can experience all of the major complications of surgery during and after operations and, depending on their overall medical status, may have these complications more frequently and to a more severe degree. Thus, preoperative evaluation should include not only the tumor type and stage of disease but also the general medical status of the patient.

The postoperative recovery environment and length of time should be clearly established before the procedure is undertaken. If the patient is likely to have a long recovery period with only a short hospitalization with intensive nursing, then appropriate plans must be made for care in the home or another outpatient setting.

The Principles of Operating for Advanced Cancer

- The site of the incision is crucial. A poorly placed incision can compromise an otherwise successful operation. Incisions in patients with advanced cancer may heal slowly. Incisions should be placed where they provide good access and healing. Some incision sites, such as the lower midline abdomen, are notoriously poor at healing and should be avoided. In a similar fashion, prior areas of radiation therapy are not desirable sites for incision placement.
- Each patient must undergo the procedure that is optimal for him or her. The surgery is tailored to each individual patient's needs and medical status. For example, the decision to attempt a resection or bypass procedure in bowel obstruction depends on the patient's fitness and age and the available postoperative care facilities. A noncurative resection of bowel obstruction with an anastomosis and tumor removal might well be a better palliative procedure in terms of quality of life than a simple short bypass that is likely to cause additional complications or continued pain due to the presence of a tumor. The decision as to whether to resect bowel may be complicated by prior radiation therapy.

The Principles of Postoperative Care

- Optimize the recovery by avoiding complications. Postoperative complications can be avoided or minimized by good preoperative planning, especially by assuring that optimal postoperative care is available. Many patients with cancer have an impaired nutritional status, and every attempt should be made to address and correct this, if possible, before surgery.
- Early diagnosis and aggressive management of complications are important. All surgical complications can be particularly troublesome in cancer patients, including bleeding, infection, poor wound healing, electrolyte and acid-base disorders, renal failure, airway obstruction, and problems related to prolonged immobiliz-

ation (such as pressure sores, pulmonary embolus, muscle wasting, and psychologic stress from inactivity and prolonged hospitalization). Many of these complications are potentially fatal and therefore should be treated early and aggressively.

There are a paucity of scientific data and controlled clinical trials to determine the proper role of palliative surgery for advanced cancer. Surgical interventions are consequently based largely on principles, experience, and information from surgery in other settings, and new scientific investigations are required.

Indications for Surgery

As noted by Veronesi (1982), the indications for palliative surgery are less well defined than are those for curative surgery, and they must be weighed on an individual basis in the light of the rate of disease progression, the life expectancy, the seriousness of the disturbance produced by the disease, and the degree of improvement of symptoms that can be expected. As a general rule, palliative surgery is contemplated for lesions causing obstruction, compression, bleeding, pain, and other symptoms.

OBSTRUCTION

Surgical intervention for obstruction is usually directed at the gastrointestinal tract, the genitourinary tract, the bile ducts, and the blood vessels. There is rarely a need for surgery in patients with obstructions of the respiratory tract or lymphatic system.

Obstructions of the gastrointestinal tract are the ones that most often require surgical intervention. The most frequent sites are the esophagus, the gastric pylorus, the small bowel, and the distal large bowel. Patency of the esophagus can be maintained by the insertion of an intracavitary prosthesis, and pyloric obstruction can be managed by creating a gastroenteric anastomosis. When feasible, bowel obstruction is dealt with by resection, bypass, or, in the case of large bowel tumors, colostomy. An obstruction of the ureter is not uncommon in patients with pelvic tumors and may occur either unilaterally or bilaterally. The ureters can be given an outlet either on the skin or into the large intestine. Also a nephrostomy can be performed. Lower urinary tract obstruction can be managed by utilizing a cystostomy.

Tumors causing obstruction of a bile duct are usually cancers of the head of the pancreas or, more rarely, metastatic lymph nodes of the porta hepatis. In these instances, good palliation can be achieved by diversion of the bile flow into the jejunum or stomach.

Finally, operations for arterial occlusion are rare but may be necessary, as in the case of occlusion of the common carotid artery by metastases from head and neck cancers.

COMPRESSION OF THE SPINAL CORD

Approximately half of the patients with compression of the spinal cord have advanced disease with metastases (Forbes 1988). The early diagnosis of this problem is important to prevent the tragedy of a patient with permanent paraplegia. Although opinions differ as to the exact role and timing of surgery (decompressive laminectomy) and radiation therapy, procrastination is to be avoided.

Sorensen et al. (1990), in a seven-year retrospective review, studied the outcome of 345 patients treated for metastatic spinal core compression with radiation therapy alone, laminectomy alone, or laminectomy followed by radiation therapy. Carcinomas of the lung, prostate, breast, and kidney were the commonest malignant neoplasms causing cord compression. The outcome of therapy depended primarily on the patient's ambulatory status at the time of the diagnosis. The majority of the patients (79 percent) who were able to walk before treatment remained ambulatory, in contrast to the 21 percent of the nonambulatory paraplegic patients and the 6 percent of the paralytic patients who regained walking ability. Patients managed with laminectomy followed by radiation therapy responded better than did patients treated with radiation therapy or laminectomy alone; when the patient's pretreatment motor status was considered, however, there was no significant difference among the three forms of therapy. In the subgroup of nonambulatory patients, however, a significantly better restoration of gait was observed in patients treated with combined laminectomy and radiation therapy than in patients treated with radiation therapy alone. The median survival of all patients was 3.1 months. The results of this study, as suggested by the investigators, point out the need for a prospective, randomized study to answer the question as to which modality or combination is optimal for the treatment of metastatic compression of the spinal cord.

BLEEDING

Although it would be distinctly unusual, surgery can play a vital role in the management of bleeding problems. Bleeding from gastric infiltration from advanced lymphoma or carcinoma may require gastric resection if nonsurgical measures are not successful (Veronesi 1982). As noted previously, explosive bleeding from tumor erosion into the carotid artery may require surgical intervention.

PAIN

Neurosurgical procedures can play an important part in managing pain. This will be discussed in part II.

FRACTURE

Surgery is indicated for patients with metastatic bone disease causing pathologic fractures and pain. The aims of this orthopedic intervention are to control pain and preserve remaining function so patients can be mobilized.

Bono et al. (1991) reported the results of palliative surgery for metastatic bone disease performed during a 10-year period. Among 349 patients with bone metastases, 83 (24 percent) required one or more surgical procedures. The commonest tumor sites were breast, lung, prostate, and kidney. A variety of orthopedic procedures were employed. Of the total of 83 patients with metastatic bone disease, surgery was done in 19 patients at the prefracture stage, in 54 cases after complete fracture, and in 10 patients to decompress the spinal cord. Positive short-term results were obtained in more than 75 percent of the patients, with a mean survival time of 11.4 months. Seven patients developed mild complications. Surgical intervention is considered if metastatic bone pain is not relieved by other means; if fracture is imminent, as indicated by the loss of more than half of the cortical bone thickness; or if a fracture has already occurred (Editorial 1992).

OTHER SYMPTOMS

Dramatic as it sounds, amputation is occasionally a useful operation for patients with advanced cancer. Specifically, it is indicated in peripheral solid and bone tumors that are unresponsive to radiation therapy and are painful, are in danger of fungation, or grossly interfere with function by virtue of bulk (Philips 1984).

Patients requiring multiple paracenteses for recurrent malignant ascites may be candidates for the placement of a peritoneovenous shunt (LeVeen or Denver shunt). Although the concept of returning ascitic fluid to the intravascular space in not new, recent improvements in technology with peritoneovenous devices have led to their widespread use. These devices consist of a length of multiply perforated tube inserted in the peritoneal cavity, a length of tubing placed into the superior vena cava or the right atrium, and a unidirectional flow valve connecting the two arms (Baker 1989). The main difference between the LeVeen and Denver shunts is the one-way valve in the Denver shunt that can be manually pumped to flush any accumulated debris at periodic intervals. Despite this theoretical advantage of the Denver shunt, clinically there is no difference in the effectiveness of the two shunts.

Baker (1989) summarized the results of 15 reported studies involving 372 patients managed by the placement of a peritoneovenous shunt to control malignant ascites. The majority of patients had ovarian, gastrointestinal, or breast cancer. The median survivals ranged from 5 to 16 weeks, with 0 to 12 percent alive at one year. Response to shunting varied from 32 to 100 percent, with most studies reporting good to excellent relief of symptoms.

Summary

Palliative surgery, much like other modalities of controlling pain and symptoms, plays an important role in the medical management of dying patients. Basic principles relevant to surgery have been delineated (see Table 5.1). Indications are less well defined for palliative surgery than for curative surgery and must be individualized. In general, contemplate palliative surgery for lesions causing obstruction, compression of the spinal cord, bleeding, pain (see part II), fracture, and other symptoms. Prospective clinical trials are needed to define clearly the role of palliative surgery in patients with advanced cancer.

PART II

The Management of Pain

Chapter 6

An Overview of Pain Management

Recent publicity regarding euthanasia (Humphry 1991; Kevorkian 1991) has clearly focused for the medical community the issue of pain control in the dying patient. Existing information suggests that one-third of cancer patients undergoing active treatment and 60 to 90 percent of patients with advanced disease experience moderate to severe pain (Foley 1985). In addition, some 20 to 50 percent of patients with all stages of cancer have pain severe enough to be treated with opioid analgesics (Portenoy 1990).

The Principles of Pain Management

Certain general principles are important in the evaluation of a patient's complaint of pain. Failure to follow these principles is a major cause for poor pain control.

- Believe the patient's complaint of pain. On occasion, it is necessary to ask family members or other caregivers to corroborate the patient's report of pain. When there is doubt, trust the patient.

    Ask the patient to assess the severity of the pain using pain intensity scales. These scales often use word descriptions (0 = "no pain" to 4 = "excruciating pain") or visual analogs (a horizontal line starting with "no pain" and ending with "worst pain") whereby the patient indicates his or her perception of the pain (fig. 6.1).

    In addition to the visual analog scales, several other, more sophisticated instruments are available to measure pain. The McGill Pain Questionnaire (MPQ) is one of the most widely used tools for assessing pain. It instructs patients to make relevant selections from a list of 78 adjectives used to describe pain. An analysis of a patient's response helps the physician to determine the extent to which the pain is mainly sensory, affective, or evaluative. The

Visual Analog Scale

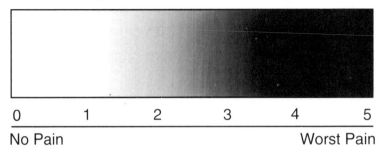

0   1   2   3   4   5

No Pain   Worst Pain

Figure 6.1 A Visual Analog Scale for Assessing Pain

MPQ also provides a schematic body figure, which the patient shades to indicate where the pain is located. Other more practical and clinically useful tools for assessing pain include the (Wisconsin) Brief Pain Inventory (BPI) and the Memorial Pain Assessment Card (MPAC). The BPI is self-administered and requires little time to complete. Features of the BPI include graphic representation of the location of the pain, groups of qualitative descriptors, visual analog scales to measure the severity of the pain, and a perceived level of interference with normal function. The MPAC is a simple, efficient, and valid pain assessment instrument that provides rapid clinical evaluation. Scales for quantifying the intensity of the pain, relief from pain, and mood and a set of descriptive adjectives are part of the MPAC. The MPAC is intended to help physicians distinguish the intensity of the pain, relief, and psychologic distress (Rowlingson, Hamill, and Patt 1993). Physicians often tend to underestimate the patient's perception of pain (Peteet et al. 1986).
• Elicit a careful history of the pain. Inquire as to when the pain occurs; its intensity, duration, character, and anatomic site(s); and precipitating and alleviating factors. The intensity of pain is quantified using one of the previously described pain intensity scales by the physicians and caregivers. In this fashion, serial scores can determine objective changes in the patient's perception of pain as various therapeutic maneuvers are tried.
• Assess for psychologic and social factors confounding the patient's expression of pain. For example, certain cultures stress the importance of stoicism, and patients steeped in those cultures rarely complain of pain, since this is viewed as a weakness. Other major impediments to good pain control are social factors, a common one being the family-patient dynamics regarding the ownership of

pain. Failure to recognize this problem often results in convoluted and fragmented pain management. Avoidance of this is best accomplished by remembering the first principle: believe the patient's complaint of pain.

- Perform a careful medical and neurologic examination in addition to reviewing the results of various diagnostic procedures. The wizardry of modern medical technology notwithstanding, bedside examination of the patient is critical in diagnosing the cause of pain. Understanding the limits of the diagnostic procedures is also important. To illustrate, in patients with multiple myeloma, the bone scan is often normal, whereas the bone survey frequently demonstrates the presence of osteolytic bone lesions.
- Evaluate the extent of the disease. Patients with advanced disease, regardless of the cause, are more apt to have pain-related problems than are those with earlier disease.
- Manage the pain symptoms during the assessment to facilitate the diagnostic work-up. Allowing patients to suffer from pain during evaluation procedures is no longer acceptable. Patients may experience pain during the evaluation and also often be subjected to additional discomfort as part of the work-up (procedure pain). This procedure pain, in turn, acts as another complicating variable. In addition, a placebo should not be used to expedite the evaluation of pain.
- Diagnose the cause of the pain and then outline and initiate a therapeutic approach. Pain is a symptom, not a diagnosis. Thus, it is critical to delineate the underlying cause of the pain. Once this step is accomplished, a therapeutic approach is outlined and started. To prevent potential conflict, it is extremely important that the patient and family agree with this approach.
- Assess pain continuously with treatment. As previously noted, the use of a pain assessment instrument, by both the patient and the caregiver, is very helpful in measuring the effects of the therapeutic interventions.

Finally, pain assessment is an ongoing, continuous process. The causes of pain often change in a patient during the course of the disease, frequently necessitating a change in treatment.

The Ladder Approach

The World Health Organization (WHO) Cancer Pain Relief program has advocated the use of an analgesic ladder as a guide to the management of cancer pain (Ventafridda et al. 1987). This approach starts with nonopioid drugs, such as acetaminophen and the nonsteroidal anti-inflammatory drugs, for mild to moderate pain. If the pain persists, the next step is to use a weak opioid, like codeine or oxycodone. If no pain relief is obtained, use a strong opioid, morphine. (Patients with severe pain go straight to the top of the ladder for treatment with a strong opioid.) At each step of the ladder, adjuvant analgesics may be used (fig. 6.2).

The WHO ladder provides a rational and logical approach to pain management, and it is applicable not only to cancer but also to all areas where pain control is needed.

The Use of Nonopioid Analgesics

Nonopioid analgesics are the first-line agents for the management of mild to moderate pain. This group includes acetaminophen and the nonsteroidal anti-inflammatory drugs (NSAIDs), such as aspirin, ibuprofen, fenoprofen, and naproxen (table 6.1). These drugs are commonly used orally; tolerance and physical dependence do not occur with repeated administration. However, the analgesic effectiveness of the nonopioid drugs is limited by a ceiling effect, that is, escalation of the dosage beyond a certain level does not produce additional analgesia. This ceiling is usually identified by slow escalation of the dosage and may vary from patient to patient. Guidelines, which are largely empiric, for the use of NSAIDs follow.

- Select the drug. NSAIDs are useful for mild to moderate pain and often provide additive analgesia when combined with opioids in

```
                                                   STRONG OPIOID ± NONOPIOID
                                                  ┌───────────────────────────
                                                  │        ± ADJUVANT
                          WEAK OPIOID ± NONOPIOID │
                         ┌────────────────────────┘
                         │       ± ADJUVANT
          NONOPIOID      │
         ┌───────────────┘
         │ ± ADJUVANT
```

Figure 6.2   The World Health Organization Analgesic Ladder

Table 6.1 The Nonopioid Analgesics

Drug	Half-life (h)	Starting Oral Dose (mg/24h)	Maximum Oral Dose (mg/24h)	Duration of Effect (h)
p-Aminophenol derivatives				
Acetaminophen[a]	2–4	1,400	6,000[e]	4–6
Salicylates				
Aspirin	3–5	1,400	6,000[e]	4–6
Diflunisal	8–12	1,000 as loading dose, then 500 every 12h	1,500	8–12
Choline magnesium trisalicylate[a]	9–17	1,500 as loading dose, then 1,000 every 12h	4,000	8–12
Salsalate[a]	8–12	1,500 as loading dose, then 1,000 every 12h	4,000	8–12
Propionic acids				
Ibuprofen	1.8–2.5	1,200	4,200[e]	4–6
Naproxen	12–15	500	1,000	≤7
Naproxen sodium	12–15	550	1,100	≤7
Fenoprofen	2–3	800	3,200	4–6
Ketoprofen	2–4	150	300	6–8
Indoles				
Indomethacin	4.5–6	75	200	4–6
Tolmetin	1–1.5	600	2,000	6–8
Sulindac	8–16	300	400	8–12
Fenamates				
Mefenamic acid[b]	2–4	500 as loading dose, then 250 every 6h	1,000	6
Meclofenamate	0.5–2	150	400	6–8
Oxicams				
Piroxicam[c]	0–86	20	40[e]	48–72
Pyrazoles				
Phenylbutazone[d]	50–100	300	400	6–8

Source: Enck (1992).

[a]Fewer gastrointestinal and hematologic side effects.

[b]Not recommended for use more than one week; therefore, not appropriate for chronic pain management.

[c]Dose of 40 mg/day for three weeks is associated with a high incidence of peptic ulcer, especially in older patients.

[d]Associated with the risk of severe marrow suppression and not preferred for chronic pain treatment.

[e]Doses that exceed the recommended daily dose may be necessary in some cases.

the treatment of severe pain. They may be especially useful for patients with bone pain or pain associated with inflammatory lesions. Gastrointestinal irritation and ulceration as well as bleeding due to platelet dysfunction are the best-known toxicities associated with NSAIDs. Often these side effects limit the clinical utility of NSAIDs for the management of chronic pain.

• Investigate the dose-response relationship. Doses of NSAIDs should initially be low and then slowly be increased, at weekly intervals, to try to identify the ceiling dose. For older patients, the starting dose should be one-half to two-thirds the recommended dose. The lack of further analgesia after a dose increment suggests that the ceiling has been reached, and the dose can be lowered to the previous level. Because of the dose-related toxicity of the NSAIDs, a maximal dose of 1.5 to 2 times the standard recommended dose is suggested in exploring the dose-response curve.

• Determine the length of the trial. In chronic cancer pain, the trial duration is usually a week or two; however, for other chronic diseases it sometimes takes weeks of treatment to determine the efficacy.

• Change to another NSAID if necessary. Because of individual variation, if one NSAID does not produce adequate analgesia, try another. Before changing to a different NSAID, it is critical that the clinician ensure that the patient has been compliant in taking the drug.

The Use of Opioid Analgesics

After the ceiling effect is reached, drug-related toxicity occurs, or disease progression is evident by changing pain control, the opioid analgesics are the next step. These drugs, used for moderate to severe pain, are characterized by their complex interaction with multiple nervous system opioid receptors. The opioid-agonist drugs, such as morphine, bind to specific opioid receptors, producing analgesia. The opioid-antagonist drugs block the effect of morphine at its receptor. Between these two groups are the mixed agonist-antagonist drugs, which, depending on the circumstances, demonstrate either agonist or antagonist properties (tables 6.2 and 6.3).

The morphinelike agonists are the most widely used drugs to manage cancer pain. Of the opioids, oral morphine is the drug of choice. Although meperidine is a morphinelike agonist, it is not appropriate for the chronic treatment of cancer pain. Long-term administration of meperidine results in the accumulation of its metabolite, norme-

Table 6.2 The Pharmacologic Effects of the Opioids at Receptor Sites

Mu Receptor	Kappa Receptor	Sigma Receptor
Supraspinal analgesia	Spinal analgesia	Dysphoria
Respiratory depression	Miosis	Psychomotor stimulation
Euphoria	Marked sedation	Hallucinations
Physical dependence		
Moderate sedation		

Sources: Lindley, Dalton, and Fields (1990); Lipman (1989).

Table 6.3 The Relative Activities of the Opioids at Receptor Sites

Drug	Mu Receptor	Kappa Receptor	Sigma Receptor
Morphinelike agonists	High activity	Moderate activity	Minimal to no activity
Mixed agonists-antagonists	No activity	High to moderate activity	High to low activity
Partial agonists	Moderate activity	Minimal activity	Minimal to no activity
Antagonist	High activity	High activity	Minimal activity

Sources: Lindley, Dalton, and Fields (1990); Lipman (1989).

peridine, which causes central nervous system excitation (Lipman 1989). Also, care must be taken when using methadone. Because of its long half-life (15 to 30 hours), chronic methadone dosing can lead to drug accumulation with the clinical results of oversedation and, rarely, coma.

The mixed agonist-antagonist drugs produce analgesia in the non-tolerant patient but will precipitate withdrawal in patients tolerant to morphinelike drugs. Therefore, when these drugs are used, they should be tried before the repeated administration of an opioid agonist. Because the incidence and severity of psychotomimetic side effects increase with escalation of the dosage and because only pentazocine is available in an oral preparation, these drugs play a very limited role in the management of chronic pain.

The partial agonist buprenorphine also may precipitate withdrawal in patients tolerant to morphinelike agonists and, like the mixed agonist-antagonist, should be used before using the opioid-like agonist. Unlike the mixed agonist-antagonists, buprenorphine does not cause the psychotomimetic side effects. However, buprenorphine is available only in a parenteral form.

Guidelines for the use of opioid analgesics, which stress the individualization of therapy, follow:

- Avoid dosing "as needed" (prn). Dosing "as needed" (prn) causes a "peak and trough" effect on the blood levels of the drug, which results in uneven analgesia (fig. 6.3). Round-the-clock dosing, on the other hand, provides a constant, unfluctuating blood level of the analgesic (fig. 6.4). Start with the lowest possible dose and titrate upward.
- Know the pharmacology of the drug used. Select and be comfortable with the use of one or two opioids. See table 6.4 for details relating to the pharmacology of the opioids.
- Choose the route of administration to maximize the analgesic effect. The oral route is preferred for overall convenience and comfort, but occasionally other routes, such as parenteral, mucosal, intrathecal, or transdermal, are necessary.
- Use drug combinations to enhance analgesia. Combinations providing additive analgesia may reduce side effects and limit the dose escalation of the opioid component in the combination. For example, codeine combined with acetaminophen provides effective additive analgesia.
- Avoid drug combinations that increase sedation without enhanc-

PRN (as needed)

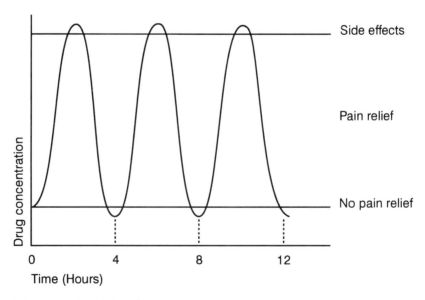

Figure 6.3   Dosing "as Needed" (prn)

Round the Clock

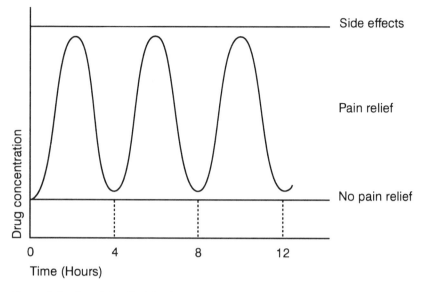

Figure 6.4 Round-the-Clock Dosing

ing analgesia. The empiric use of phenothiazines with morphine, for example, should be avoided.

- Anticipate, recognize, and treat side effects appropriately. Side effects of opioids are either central nervous system (CNS) related (sedation, nausea and vomiting, agitation, respiratory depression) or not CNS related (dry mouth, constipation, sweating, itching, urinary retention).
- Watch for the development of tolerance, and manage appropriately. Tolerance, or the need for escalating doses of opioids to maintain adequate analgesia, seems to occur in all patients receiving opioids chronically. Treat the patient who develops tolerance by switching to an alternative opioid analgesic. Due to incomplete cross-tolerance, patients who become tolerant to one opioid can be switched to another opioid to provide better analgesia. One-half of the calculated equianalgesic dose of the new drug is recommended in titrating the initial dose.
- Prevent acute withdrawal. Acute withdrawal is prevented by tapering the drugs slowly and using naloxone cautiously in patients on chronic opioids.
- Respect and expect individual differences in pain and response to

Table 6.4   The Opioid Analgesics

Drug	Equianalgesic Dose (mg)	Half-life (h)	Starting Oral Dose (mg)	Peak Effect (h)[c]	Duration (h)
Morphinelike agonists					
Morphine	10 IM[a]	2–3	30–60[b]	0.5–1.0	3–6
	60 PO[b]			1.5–2.0	4–7
Controlled-release morphine	20–60 PO	2–3	60–90	3–4	8–12
Hydromorphone	1.5 IM	2–3	4–8	0.5–1.0	3–4
	7.5 PO			1–2	3–4
Oxymorphone	1 IM	2–3	—	0.5–1	3–6
	10 PR			1.5–3	4–6
Methadone	10 IM	15–30	5–10	0.5–1.5	4–6
	20 PO			1.5–2.0	6–8
Meperidine	75 IM	2–3	75	0.5–1	3–4
	300 PO			1–2	3–6
Levorphanol	2 IM	12–16	2–4	0.5–1.0	4–6
	4 PO			1.5–2.0	4–7
Codeine	130 IM	2–3	60	1.5–2.0	3–6
	200 PO				
Oxycodone	15 IM	2–3	5	1	3–6
	30 PO				
Hydrocodone	Available only in combination	2–4	—	0.5–1	3–4
Propoxyphene HCl	130 PO	12	65–130	1.5–2	3–6
Propoxyphene naprylate	130 PO	12	65–130	1.5–2	3–6
Mixed agonists-antagonists					
Pentazocine	60 IM	2–3	30–60	0.5–1	3–6
	180 PO			1–2	3–6
Nalbuphine	10 IM	4–6	Not available	0.5–1	3–6
Butorphanol	2 IM	2–3	Not available	0.5–1	3–4
Partial agonists					
Buprenorphine	0.4 IM	2–5	Not available	0.5–1	4–6
	0.8 SL			2–3	5–6

Source: Enck (1992).

[a]Morphine, 10 mg IM, is the standard of comparison for equianalgesia. IM, intramuscular; PO, per os; PR, per rectum; SL, sublingual.

[b]Relative potency of IM:PO morphine is 1:6 for acute pain. This ratio changes to 1:2–3 with chronic dosing.

[c]Onset of action of these drugs is generally 15 to 30 minutes.

therapy. Older patients are more sensitive to the opioid analgesics and respond to morphine as though they had received three or four times the normal dose given to younger patients (Kaiko et al. 1982). Also, older patients are more susceptible to the side effects of both the NSAIDs and the opioids.

The Use of Adjuvant Analgesic Drugs

Adjuvant analgesic agents represent the third group of drugs used to treat chronic pain. These drugs produce analgesia by mechanisms not clearly known and not directly related to the opioid receptor system. Adjuvant analgesics include anticonvulsants, phenothiazines, antidepressants, antihistamines, steroids, and antibiotics (table 6.5). The benzodiazepines and cocaine do not provide additive analgesic effect to patients receiving opioids. Guidelines for the use of adjuvant analgesics follow.

- Choose a drug to match the clinical indication. The anticonvulsants, phenytoin and carbamazepine, and the tricyclic antidepressants (TCAs) are useful in managing pain of neuropathic origin, such as postherpetic neuralgia and brachial and lumbosacral plexopathy. Methotrimeprazine, a phenothiazine, produces significant analgesia independent of the opioid receptors and, therefore, does not cause significant constipation and respiratory depression. Because of these properties, methotrimeprazine is helpful in patients tolerant to opioids. Also, intermittent methotrimeprazine is useful for pain control in patients with intestinal obstruction in whom opioids only add to the problem of obstruction. Steroids, predominantly dexamethasone, are indicated for the relief of pain due to nervous system involvement by tumor. Examples of this include brain metastases, spinal cord compression, and peripheral nerve or plexus infiltration with tumor. Finally, antibiotics may aid pain relief in certain clinical situations, most notably head and neck tumors with ulcerating tumors and pain (Bruera and MacDonald 1986).
- Understand the drug and dosage. Analgesia, for example, occurs with the TCAs at a lower dose than needed for the mood-elevating effect.
- Be aware of new or heightened side effects. Dry mouth and confusion can occur with use of the TCAs. These complications are also commonly encountered in patients receiving opioids.
- Use adjuvant analgesic drugs for a finite period. Antibiotics

Table 6.5   The Adjuvant Analgesic Drugs

Drug	Starting Oral Dose (mg/24hr)	Indications for Use
Anticonvulsants		
Phenytoin[a]	100 initially, then slowly titrated to 300	Neuropathic pain, such as postherapetic neuralgia
Carbamazepine[a]	100 initially, then increased to 800 over a period of 7–10 days	Neuropathic pain
Phenothiazines		
Methotrimeprazine	Not available orally 5–15 IM[b]	Opioid-tolerant patients or to avoid opioid-induced constipation or respiratory depression
Antidepressants		
Amitriptyline	10 for older patients (25 for others), then slowly increased to 50–75 at bedtime	Neuropathic pain
Antihistamines		
Hydroxyzine[c]	25–100	Additive analgesia in combination with opioid
Steroids		
Dexamethasone	16	Nervous system involvement with or compression by tumor
Antibiotics[d]	—[d]	Acute infection associated with malignant ulceration

Source: Enck (1992).
[a]The minimal effective dose for analgesia is not known.
[b]Methotrimeprazine, 15 mg IM, is equivalent to morphine, 10 mg IM.
[c]Anecdotal observation of usefulness based on clinical practice.
[d]Depending on organism identified and/or empiric trial.

should be stopped after the signs of acute infection have resolved, generally in one to two weeks. Likewise, TCAs should be discontinued after a trial of four to six weeks if no pain-relieving effect is evident.

Managing the Complications of Pain Treatment

All three groups of drug (nonopioid, opioid, and adjuvant analgesic) used to treat chronic pain have the potential to produce clinically significant side effects.

- Be proactive rather than reactive. Constipation is a frequent problem with the use of opioid analgesics. Therefore, when a patient is started on an opioid, a bowel regimen such as a daily stool softener and laxative should also be commenced to lessen this side effect.
- Recognize and treat side effects appropriately. The major central nervous system effect of the opioids is sedation or drowsiness. This may be managed by reducing the drug dosage and prescribing the drug more frequently or by switching to an analgesic with a shorter half-life. Generally, amphetamines are not useful for enhancing the comfort of terminally ill patients. In some instances, however, they are able to decrease sedation and increase activity by offsetting the opioid side effects (Bruera, Chadwick, Brenneis, et al. 1987). Nausea and vomiting are managed by either changing the patient to an alternative opioid or using an antiemetic, such as a phenothiazine or an antihistamine. In some instances, tolerance to nausea develops and the antiemetics can be tapered. As previously mentioned, these drugs, especially the phenothiazines, can potentiate the sedating effect of the opioids.

  Respiratory depression is potentially the most serious side effect of opioid therapy. It usually occurs with the acute administration of morphine to an opioid-naive patient. Rarely, patients being treated chronically with opioids develop respiratory depression; slowly give diluted naloxone (an opioid antagonist) intravenously, and titrate carefully to prevent the precipitation of acute withdrawal symptoms.
- Prevent acute opioid withdrawal. Physical dependence is a pharmacologic effect of opioids. Withdrawal symptoms occur when the drug is stopped and are prevented by slowly tapering the drug over the course of one to two weeks. As noted above, naloxone should be used carefully in patients treated with opioids on a chronic basis.
- Avoid polypharmacy. For example, the use of steroids with the NSAIDs has the serious potential to increase not only gastrointestinal irritation but also the risk for bleeding. Confusion and other CNS toxicities are seen not only with the opioids but also with the NSAIDs and some adjuvant analgesics. Exercise care to avoid additive side effects due to the indiscriminate combination of these drugs.
- Consider alternative pain control therapies if side effects are unmanageable or intolerable. If the pain is not relieved pharmacologically, consider other therapeutic interventions.

Summary

Guidelines on evaluating a patient's complaint of pain; on the use of nonopioid, opioid, and adjuvant analgesic drugs; and on managing the complications of pain treatment are readily available to physicians. No new drugs or treatment methods are needed, only enlightenment and further education by physicians, to provide good-quality care to dying patients. Past concerns about addicting patients to opioid analgesics are scientifically unfounded. Using appropriate doses of opioid analgesics, such as morphine, for the severe pain of cancer and other chronic diseases is simply good care.

Chapter 7

Opioids

Oral Morphine

Of all natural and synthetic opioids, oral morphine is the standard for comparison and is the drug of choice for chronic severe pain. Orally administered morphine is subject to the first-pass effect of liver metabolism (glucuronidation), which causes a large reduction in its potency. In a single-dose study, Sawe et al. (1981) investigated the kinetics of both oral and intravenous morphine in seven cancer patients. They found a 15 to 64 percent variation in oral bioavailability, with a mean of 38 percent. In addition, they showed a marked interindividual variation in the terminal half-life, from 58 to 467 minutes. This unique wide individual variation in the metabolism of morphine accounts for the broad therapeutic dose range, which may vary from only 30 mg a day to several grams a day to achieve good relief of pain (Hoskin and Hanks 1990).

The intramuscular administration of morphine at a dose of 10 mg is considered the standard for comparison to other dosages and other opioid analgesics. Morphine given in this manner and dose produces an onset of action at 20 to 60 minutes, with a peak effect at 30 to 60 minutes and a three- to six-hour duration. For a similar but slightly larger effect, the oral dose is 60 mg for acute pain and 20 to 30 mg for chronic administration (Berry 1988). This difference in oral:parenteral potency from 6:1 in acute dosing versus 2–3:1 for chronic dosing is thought to be due to the accumulation of the pharmacologically active metabolite morphine-6-glucuronide (Weissman, Dahl, and Joranson 1990).

Clinically, the use of oral morphine remains empiric. The usual starting dosage in an opioid-naive patient is 20 to 30 mg every four hours. The most important factor determining the dose required is the severity of the pain. As reported by Hoskin and Hanks (1990), a retrospective analysis of clinical data from cancer patients indicates that age is also a predictor of dose, with patients under 60 years having a median maximum (four hourly) dose requirement of 55 mg, compared with only 25 to 30 mg for those over 60 years. Pharmacokinetic differences for morphine in different age groups have been found, with a reduced clearance and smaller volume of distribution in older patients. Other potential dose-modifying factors, such as impaired hepatic and renal functions, have not shown a significant relationship to the dosage, although pharmacokinetic studies in noncancer patients have demonstrated impaired clearance in hepatic failure and the accumulation of active metabolites in renal failure. Similarly, factors affecting the enterohepatic circulation of morphine, such as cholestasis, bowel resection, and the use of antibiotics, have not shown a meaningful effect on the overall dose requirements.

After the pain has been controlled and a 24-hour dosage of morphine has been determined, treatment can be continued with an immediate-release preparation (4-hour dosing) alone. Alternatively, a long-acting/controlled-release preparation (12-hour dosing) can be started using an immediate-release morphine for breakthrough pain.

Controlled-release Oral Morphine

Although controlled-release oral morphine preparations have been available in the United States for some time, the use of these products has been a source of confusion and misunderstanding by caregivers, especially physicians. This problem was highlighted in a recent study by White et al. (1991), who sought to assess prescribing practices for patients with cancer pain among populations of physicians in the United Kingdom. A postal questionnaire was sent to every member of the medical staff in four different types of medical practice to try to provide a broad view of physicians' attitudes. These practices included a specialist oncology hospital, an undergraduate teaching hospital, a general hospital, and general practitioners in both inner city and suburban areas.

Overall, the response rate to the questionnaire was 42 percent (265/625). The drug of first choice for analgesia in patients with severe cancer pain was morphine; it was chosen by 66 percent of physicians. Further analysis of this group showed that 20 percent prescribed a morphine elixir and 46 percent preferred a controlled-release morphine (MST Continus) preparation. The use of this controlled-release product was particularly popular among general practitioners and younger physicians. MST was also chosen by 56 percent of physicians with no oncology experience but by only 30 percent of those with more than three years experience in oncology.

The vast majority of respondents (93 percent) indicated that they would administer their drug of first choice regularly, and 84 percent chose the oral route as their first choice of administration. Of the physicians who preferred MST, 63 percent would administer the drug at 12-hour intervals, whereas 37 percent indicated that they would use the drug at less than 12-hour intervals. Of the entire group of responding physicians, only 17 percent choosing morphine defined an upper dose limit; of these, 12 percent used MST as the preferred formulation.

In this study, most physicians chose morphine as their first-choice analgesic, 84 percent chose the oral route, and 87 percent indicated that they would administer the analgesic on a regular basis. Morphine elixir was the formulation of choice in the specialist oncology hospital, but controlled-release morphine tablets (MST) were the preferred form in both other hospitals and general practice. MST was clearly preferred by those with less than five years of experience. MST was prescribed in regimens varying from once a day to every 2 hours. As noted by the authors, this indicates considerable confusion about controlled-release morphine. Although the awareness of the preparation is very high, the drug seems to be subject to widespread misuse. MST is designed for 12-hourly administration and infrequently has to be given more often.

A well-known principle in the use of morphine for pain due to advanced cancer is that there is no arbitrary upper limit of the dose, since morphine has no ceiling effect. A minority of the respondents in this study did indicate an upper dose limit and, in many cases, at a fairly modest level. It is notable that the majority of these physicians used MST as their preferred formulation. There is little doubt that, if this survey were done in the United States, similar misperceptions regarding controlled-release morphine preparations would be identified in U.S. physicians.

Because oral morphine has a short half-life, peak effect, and duration, it must be administered every four hours to achieve optimal effect. Unfortunately, a four-hour regimen is inconvenient for patients because it requires dosing during the night. In addition, compliance is known to decrease as the required frequency of dosing increases, and noncompliance adds to the risk of suboptimal pain control.

In a study of pharmacokinetics and clinical efficacy, Thirlwell et al. (1989) compared an oral morphine solution given every 4 hours to a controlled-release morphine table (MS Contin) administered every 12 hours in 23 adult patients with chronic pain due to cancer. The steady-state plasma concentration versus time profile obtained in cancer patients taking MS Contin every 12 hours demonstrated that the prolonged release of morphine from tablets reduced both the rate of absorption and the rate of decline of plasma morphine concentrations. As suggested by the authors, these pharmacokinetics indicate that a 12-hour regimen of MS Contin should be optimal for most patients. Although plasma concentrations of morphine were declining at the end of the 12-hour period, at no time did they fall significantly below the corresponding concentrations achieved with the morphine solution. This finding parallels the clinical observation that there is no loss of analgesic efficacy over the last few hours of the MS Contin dose interval.

Furthermore, Thirlwell et al. (1989) confirmed what others (Hanks 1989) had reported, namely, that 12-hour dosing with controlled-release morphine produces pain control equivalent to that achieved with a 4-hour regimen. They also suggested a daily milligram equivalency when transferring patients from oral morphine preparations to controlled-release formulations such as MS-Contin.

Clearly, controlled-release morphine is for maintenance treatment once the patient's morphine requirement has been determined, and it is inappropriate for administration "as required." The pattern of adverse effects with these formulations seems to be similar to that of conventional oral morphine preparations. However, there may be some advantage in the quality of sleep with controlled-release morphine, possibly related to fewer fluctuations in plasma and central nervous system concentrations of morphine and its metabolites (Hanks 1989).

Parenteral Opioids

Treatment with parenteral opioids is especially useful in patients who cannot tolerate the oral route. Studies of pain management show that the majority of patients require at least two routes of administration (oral and parenteral) during the course of their painful disease and that one-third require at least three alternative routes (Coyle et al. 1990).

CONTINUOUS INTRAVENOUS INFUSIONS

The continuous intravenous infusion of opioid analgesics has been used in the management of both postoperative pain and chronic cancer pain. One study of 210 dying patients treated during a two-year period revealed that 13 percent received a continuous intravenous infusion of morphine before death (Kellar 1984). In 1986, Portenoy et al. published the results of a three-year retrospective review of their experience with continuous intravenous infusions in hospitalized cancer patients of the Pain Service at Memorial Sloan-Kettering Cancer Center. Forty-six infusions in 36 patients were identified for study. These 46 infusions accounted for approximately 3 percent of Pain Service consultations during the three-year period.

The median age of the 36 patients was 42 years, with a range of 1.5 to 67 years. All patients had received opioids before starting infusions, with wide variation in the quantity of opioids consumed during the 24 hours preceding the infusions. Morphine was the most frequently infused drug (36 patients), followed by methadone (4), hydromorphone (4), oxymorphone (1), and levorphanol (1). In morphine equivalents, the mean starting dose was 17 mg/hour, the mean maximum infusion rate was 69 mg/hour, and the mean rate of infusion termination was 52 mg/hour. The duration of the infusions varied from 1 to 45 days.

Pain relief was defined as acceptable if the patient remained awake and coherent and analgesia was reported to be adequate in either nurse's or physician's notes during consecutive days after the infusion was started. Based on these criteria, pain was relieved in 61 percent of the patients, leaving 37 percent with inadequate pain control. Pain relief was indeterminate in one patient.

The authors were uncertain as to why more than one-third of the patients were unable to obtain adequate pain control with continuous intravenous infusion, but they offered several explanations. They noted that this phenomenon was observed most commonly in patients whose pain occurred episodically, usually with movement (incident pain), in those whose pain was due to nervous system injury that interrupted the normal transmission of sensory impulses (deafferentation pain), and in those whose pain was a component of a more global nature not amenable to treatment with opioids. Side effects were common and included sedation, confusion, nausea, and vomiting. Respiratory depression occurred in only one patient, who was also concurrently receiving intrathecal morphine. Portenoy et al. (1986) thought that the continuous intravenous infusion of opioids, predominantly morphine, was safe, but they recommended a trial of repetitive intravenous bolus dosing before initiating continuous infusion in most patients.

Based on this study, as well as others, I suggest the following indications for the use of the continuous intravenous infusion of opioids:

- intolerance of intramuscular and oral routes;
- the need for frequent injections, more often than every two hours, for pain control;

• the presence of prominent bolus effects, such as sedation or the
  rapid return of pain after injections, on repetitive dosing; and
• the need for rapid titration (Portenoy et al. 1986; Payne 1987a).

Rarely, patients require very high doses of continuous intravenous
morphine for pain control. In a five-year retrospective review, Gregory
et al. (1991) identified six patients at the Johns Hopkins Oncology
Center who were treated with more than 4 grams of intravenous morphine per day. Three patients received this dosage for less than 24
hours without seizures. Two of the three remaining patients developed
grand mal seizures on the second and third days after morphine infusions of 4.8 and 6.7 grams/day, respectively. Upon further study, the
investigators found that intravenous solutions of morphine typically
contained bisulfite preservatives. The usual exposure to these bisulfite
preservatives was less than 100 mg/day, and higher doses, especially
when given continuously, had previously been associated with seizures.
Based on this, the authors postulated that prolonged intravenous infusion of high-dose morphine places patients at risk for seizures from the
accumulation of toxic doses of bisulfite preservatives. Furthermore,
they suggested that patients requiring high doses of intravenous
opioids should receive agents that are free of bisulfite preservatives.
    Unfortunately, continuous intravenous infusions are cumbersome,
expensive, and not readily transportable to the home setting. Therefore, the use of continuous subcutaneous infusions has provided a
viable alternative.

CONTINUOUS SUBCUTANEOUS INFUSIONS

    In 1986, Coyle et al., from the Pain Service at Memorial Sloan Ket-
tering Cancer Center, reported their experience with 15 patients with
advanced cancer who were managed with the continuous subcutaneous infusion of opioids. The mean age of these patients was 54 years,
with a range of 23 to 71 years. Nine of the 15 patients had either
obstruction or a malabsorption syndrome, and all had prior treatment
with parental opioids. Morphine was the most common opioid used in
9 patients (range, 3.5 to 9.7 mg/hour), followed by hydromorphone in
3 (range, 1.0 to 7.5 mg/hour), levorphanol in 2 (range, 1.0 to 4.0
mg/hour), and methadone in 1 (range, 10.0 to 24 mg/hour). Subcutaneous infusion utilized a portable, battery-operated infusion pump
attached to a 27 gauge butterfly needle placed subcutaneously. Any
subcutaneous site could be used on a rotating basis, but the subclavicu-
lar area and anterior chest wall were frequently used to permit free
movement of the patient's extremities. The complete tubing, infusion

site, and needle were routinely changed every week. Patients remained on the continuous subcutaneous infusion for 3 to 76 days. Thirteen of the 15 patients (87 percent) rated their pain control as good. The only complication was local irritation at the infusion site in 5 patients. The average patient underwent a change of site every three days, although one patient required this every six hours (Coyle et al. 1986; Maouskop et al. 1985).

According to this group, the major indication for continuous subcutaneous infusion of opioids is the requirement for prolonged administration of parenteral opioids. Subcutaneous infusions offer the following significant advantages over the use of intermittent subcutaneous, intramuscular, or intravenous routes:

- They avoid repetitive intramuscular/subcutaneous injections.
- They avoid the need for intravenous access.
- They free the patient from delay in the administration of opioid analgesic.
- They provide a continuous level of pain control with no peak-level side effects or trough-level pain breakthrough.
- They are readily accepted and managed by patients and their families.
- They allow earlier discharge home without compromising pain control (Coyle et al. 1986; Payne 1987a).

In another study from the Cross Cancer Institute in Alberta, Canada (Bruera, Brenneis, Michaud, Chadwick, et al. 1987), 56 patients with advanced cancer were managed with continuous subcutaneous infusions of either morphine (34 patients) or hydromorphone (22 patients). Unlike the study at Memorial Sloan-Kettering Cancer Center, pain control was achieved with intravenous opioids before the start of the subcutaneous infusion. Another difference was the use of a non-battery-powered pump. The mean duration of infusion was 26 ± 14 days, with 45 percent of patients being discharged to home for an average of 18 days. After 48 hours of subcutaneous infusion, 96 percent preferred the subcutaneous infusion to their previous intravenous treatment because of increased comfort, easier mobility, and better pain control. Systemic toxicity included severe drowsiness or confusion (14 percent), which improved on adjustment of the dosage of the infusion. One patient (2 percent) developed respiratory depression, which improved with discontinuation of the hydromorphone infusion. Local toxicity consisted of infection (3 percent), chemical irritation (5 percent), and bleeding (1 percent). No difference was found between morphine and hydromorphone in pain control or toxicity. In addition, a subset of patients who were poor candidates for home discharge, namely, those requiring frequent dose increases to maintain adequate pain control, was identified. The authors of this study concluded that subcutaneous infusion of opioid with a portable disposable device is a safe and simple method for administering effective analgesia to inpatients as well as outpatients.

Few studies directly compared the subcutaneous to intravenous route of continuous infusion of opioid until the report by Moulin et al. in 1991. In a randomized, double-blind, cross-over trial, these investigators studied 53 patients with advanced cancer who had been started on continuous subcutaneous infusions of opioids because of substantial side effects from oral or rectal analgesics. Twenty patients (10 male and 10 female patients with a mean age of 62 years) participated in the study, with 23 refusing and 10 excluded because of metabolic encephalopathy or brain metastases. Using subcutaneous infusions before the trial, the investigators established the maximum analgesic dose of hydormorphone with minimal side effects. For each 48-hour trial period, new infusion sites were started on the abdomen or anterior chest wall. The study was double-blind by the use of two programmable infusion pumps. During active subcutaneous infusion, the intravenous pump delivered saline or hydomorphone. Morphine injections were given every three hours for breakthrough pain.

Serial measurements of pain intensity, pain relief, mood, and sedation using visual analog scales showed no statistically or clinically significant differences between the two routes of infusion. The mean hydromorphone infusion rate was 6.1 mg/hour, with a range of 1 to 35 mg/hour. Side effects were minimal (four patients experienced nausea). The mean number of morphine injections for breakthrough pain during the 48-hour trial period did not differ significantly between the routes (4.8 for intravenous versus 5.3 for subcutaneous). The investigators used hydromorphone because of its high analgesic potency (i.e., five to six times that of morphine). This pharmacologic property minimized the volume of infusion and maximized the duration of use of each pump reservoir. These features were particularly advantageous for the home setting of continuous subcutaneous infusions. Opioid-tolerant patients requiring more than 10 mg/hour for adequate pain control needed at least a 50-mg/hour equivalent infusion of morphine, which required a specially prepared morphine solution of high concentration or a greater volume of infusion. Because of the simplicity, technical advantages, and cost-effectiveness of continuous subcutaneous infusion of opioid, the authors advocated the abandonment of intravenous infusions for the management of severe cancer pain, except in rare circumstances.

PATIENT-CONTROLLED ANALGESIA

Some patients experience side effects related to intermittent high doses and breakthrough pain with oral opioids such as morphine. In well over half of these patients, the use of continuous intravenous or subcutaneous infusions of opioids has provided effective pain control. Therefore, the addition of a patient-controlled analgesia (PCA) system whereby patients receiving a continuous infusion of opioids could give themselves additional bolus doses was a logical extension.

PCA was initially described by Sechzer in 1968 (White 1988). At that time, he evaluated the analgesic response to small doses of intravenous opioid analgesics given on patient demand by a nurse-observer. Although this system provided improved pain relief with smaller total dosages, it proved impractical because of the demands it placed on nursing personnel.

In the late 1960s, researchers began testing instruments that would enable patients to self-administer small intravenous doses of opioids when they felt the need for them. One of the key features of these devices was the development of a lockout or delay interval. The purpose of the lockout interval was to prevent the patient from administering a second dose until after the first dose had time to exert its peak pharmacologic effect.

In 1970, investigators described an instrument that automatically administered intravenous analgesic drugs after the patient pressed the button on a handgrip device. In a pilot study involving 30 patients, they reported that patient and physician acceptance was good and that the safety features were reliable. The following year, Sechzer described his initial experience with a PCA system and concluded that it was a highly satisfactory method for treating postoperative pain and that good analgesia was achieved with relatively low total drug doses. In the ensuing years, multiple reports in the medical literature have shown the value of PCA in managing short-term, acute postoperative pain.

PCA is a system designed to accommodate a wide range of analgesic requirements. It can also minimize the anxiety resulting from the slow onset of pain relief associated with the most commonly used therapeutic modalities. A major psychologic advantage with PCA relates to its ability to minimize the time interval between the perception of pain and the administration of an analgesic. In addition, the increased attention being paid to the PCA-treated patient might provide a psychologic benefit to the patient. With PCA therapy, patients experience minimal sedation during awake hours and few side effects.

In 1986, Citron et al. published the results of their PCA study in eight patients with cancer. This open study was to determine standard dose ranges and lockout intervals in addition to patient acceptance of this mode of treatment for cancer pain. The duration of each trial was no longer than 96 hours. Respiratory rates, mental status, and pain relief were recorded at baseline and during the study period. In some patients, a loading dose of intravenous morphine was delivered by the infusion pump to provide initial pain relief. PCA doses of morphine ranged from 1 to 5 mg, with lockout intervals of 15 to 90 minutes. The length of this lockout interval was selected to prevent patients from having to self-administer medication so often that it would interfere with their activity. Many of the patients administered medication about every two hours after they achieved their initial pain control and, in general, the patients had a higher analgesic demand during the first four hours than during the remaining time of treatment. Respiratory rates decreased during the first four hours of treatment, but no cases of significant respiratory depression occurred during this period or thereafter in the study.

At the end of the study, all patients expressed satisfaction with PCA, and five patients preferred this mode of pain control over conventional methods of giving opioids. Concerns regarding potential opioid overdose with PCA therapy were addressed, and the investigators noted that proper infusion pump settings for the amount of morphine to be delivered and the lockout interval minimized this risk. Based on their study, the authors concluded that PCA was an effective and safe therapy for cancer pain.

Kerr et al. (1988) studied 18 patients with poorly controlled cancer pain who were treated with both continuous infusion (intravenous or subcutaneous) opioid therapy and PCA. This study differed from that of Citron et al. (1986) in that all patients were managed in the outpatient setting. The portable infusion pump used in the study not only administered a continuous infusion of the opioid but also permitted patients to give bolus injections "as needed."

Eighteen cancer patients completed at least one outpatient infusion of opioids. Conventional opioid dosing was changed because of breakthrough pain in most patients (15) or because of significant side effects, such as nausea and vomiting (6 patients), drowsiness (4), inconvenient frequent injection (2), and dysphagia (1). The lockout interval for the PCA was 30 to 60 minutes. Most patients received either morphine or hydromorphone. A single patient was on meperidine. The maximum dosages of these opioids were morphine, 80 mg/hour; hydromorphone, 60 mg/hour; and meperidine, 50 mg/hour. The outpatient infusions were easily manageable for long periods, with an average of 54 days and a range of 7 to 225 days. The majority of patients required some escalation of the dosage during the first 14 days. Side effects were minimal, and improved pain control was achieved by all patients.

In 1989, Swanson et al. reported the largest series of cancer patients using PCA for chronic pain. The study of these 117 patients was conducted in the setting of a private practice incorporating a community-based, multidisciplinary approach. Sixty-nine percent of the patients were treated at home, and 31 percent were managed in hospice. All patients received either a subcutaneous (87 percent) or an intravenous (13 percent) continuous infusion of opioid along with the capability of PCA bolus for breakthrough pain. There was a wide range in the amount of opioid required to achieve adequate analgesia: the patients on intravenous morphine received a larger dosage (mean of 24 mg/hour) than did those on subcutaneous infusions (mean of 6.5 mg/hour). The bolus dose of morphine was the same (4 mg) for both groups. The mean age of the patients was 61.2 years, with a preponderance of men (62 percent versus 38 percent). The vast majority of patients were treated with morphine; treatment ranged from 1 to 295 days, with an average duration of therapy of 23 days. In these patients, bone pain was the most frequent complaint.

Of the 117 patients studied, 95 percent experienced pain relief after the initiation of PCA. Side effects were rare, consisting of subcutaneous needle site infection and respiratory depression. Progressive pain due to either advancing disease or the development of drug tolerance was controlled by increasing the rates of opioid infusion. The authors concluded that continuous infusion of opioids along with PCA bolus capability can be started and administered safely in the home.

Finally, PCA may be most advantageous in the management of incident pain, that is, pain that is quiescent at rest but occurs immediately with movement. In this setting, patients can premedicate themselves on anticipation of movement. Also, gaining a sense of control, which is implicit with PCA, may be of psychologic benefit to patients.

Alternative Routes

Generally, the favored routes of administration of morphine are oral and parenteral. Alternatively, the sublingual, buccal, and rectal routes are useful (1) when oral morphine is impractical because of nausea, vomiting, bowel obstruction, or difficulty swallowing and (2) when parenteral injections are difficult or painful, as in the presence of a bleeding disorder, emaciation, or inaccessible veins.

A major advantage for the alternative routes is the avoidance of the first-pass effect, resulting in a more rapid onset and longer duration of analgesia in addition to lower doses and fewer side effects (fig. 7.1).

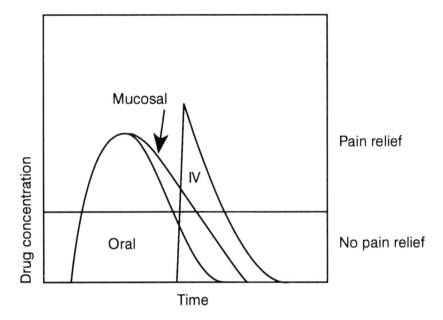

Figure 7.1   Drug Concentrations versus Time for Oral, Mucosal, and Parenteral (IV) Administrations of Morphine

However, the use of sublingual, buccal, and rectal routes can be limited by unpalatable taste and irritation of the sublingual mucosa (table 7.1).

SUBLINGUAL ADMINISTRATION

Pitorak and Kraus (1987) reported their favorable experience with sublingual morphine for pain control in hospice patients. Morphine tablets were placed sublingually. This method was preferred over the liquid preparation, since there was less likelihood that the patient would swallow the medication. Occasionally, patients complained about the bitter taste of the morphine tablet. The incidence of constipation and vomiting decreased, and pain management continued on schedule despite interruptions of gastrointestinal absorption. Lower doses of morphine were required, with a usual dosage of 10 to 40 mg every three to four hours. This lessened dose was more cost effective: a total 24-hour dose of 60 mg cost only $0.72. Despite the very limited, albeit favorable, clinical experience with the sublingual route, the question of the bioavailability of morphine is still debated (Payne 1987a).

Buprenorphine, a partial agonist with a peak and duration of effect similar to that of morphine, has also been reported as being efficacious

Table 7.1   The Advantages and Disadvantages
of Sublingual, Rectal, and Buccal Administration of Morphine

Advantages	Disadvantages
Oral or parenteral routes im-	Poor bioavailability of drugs
practicality	Unpalatable taste
Avoidance of "first pass" effects	Buccal irritation

Source: Payne (1987a).

for cancer pain control via the sublingual route. As reviewed by Payne (1987a), one study from England treated 141 cancer patients with sublingual buprenorphine in doses of 0.15 mg to 0.8 mg for an average of three months. This regimen was effective in the majority of patients, especially those with pain from head and neck cancers. Drowsiness was the commonest side effect, but dry mouth and nausea also occurred. Constipation was not seen.

BUCCAL ADMINISTRATION

Another alternative route of administering morphine is by way of the buccal mucosa membrane. Once the morphine tablet adheres to the buccal mucosa, the uptake of the active drug is principally governed by local blood flow, as with intramuscular injections. Buccal administration has advantages over sublingual drug delivery: the presence of the drug in the mouth is easily tolerated, and it does not stimulate salivation (which can speed the solution of the tablet so it is more easily swallowed and thus rendered less active).

In a study of postoperative analgesia, Bell et al. (1985) demonstrated the safety and effectiveness of buccal morphine. In this randomized study, buccal tablets containing 13.3 mg of morphine were placed between the upper lip and the gum above the incisor teeth in 20 patients. The tablets were usually moistened to facilitate their adherence to the mucosa, and they slowly dissolved within six hours. In another 20 patients, 13.3 mg of morphine was given in the form of intramuscular injection. The two routes of administration produced a similar degree of postoperative analgesia, as assessed by the average reduction in pain score and the pain relief score. Peak concentrations of plasma morphine were slightly lower after buccal than after intramuscular administration, but they declined more slowly. Consequently, the drug's bioavailability was 40 to 50 percent greater after buccal than after intramuscular administration.

The buccal route was very acceptable to patients. Only 1 of the 20 patients complained of a bitter taste and stopped the preparation after two hours. In all patients, no untoward effects on the mucosa were noted at the site of application. Nausea, vomiting, or both, as well as dizziness or drowsiness, occurred less often in the patients treated by buccal administration. Based on these findings, Bell et al. (1985) suggested that buccal morphine may be valuable in managing chronic pain due to malignant disease. Unfortunately, no large-scale study evaluating buccal morphine in this setting has been published.

RECTAL ADMINISTRATION

The third alternative for administering morphine is rectally. During a five-year period (1980–85), Steitz (1987), from Connecticut Hospice, reported an increase in the use of rectal administration from 2.2 percent (1980–81) to 6.5 percent (1984–85). This increase was attributed to better availability of suppository dosage forms of morphine.

Ellison and Lewis (1984) compared 10-mg doses of morphine in oral solution and rectal suppository in a single-dose pharmacokinetic study. They found that morphine was better absorbed from a rectal suppository than from oral solution. In addition, plasma concentrations of morphine were significantly higher during the 4.5-hour time span measured after the rectal suppository than after the oral solution. The authors stressed that these results cannot be generalized to patients receiving multiple daily doses of morphine, which is the usual clinical occurrence.

Maloney et al. (1989) described a novel use for controlled-release morphine (MS Contin) via the rectal route. All 39 of their terminally ill patients had good pain control but were unable to take oral medication because of intractable nausea, inability to swallow, or both. MS Contin 30-mg tablets were administered rectally for periods of 1 to 30 days, with a mean of 11.5 days. The dose range was 2 to 30 tablets daily, with a mean of 6.2 tablets. Sixteen patients were maintained on an every-12-hour schedule, 17 patients on an 8-hour schedule, and 6 patients on a 6-hour schedule. Pain control was maintained in all patients. In 11 patients, the dose of MS Contin was decreased. No local or systemic adverse reactions developed. In terminally ill patients, the rectal administration of tablets of MS Contin was a safe, effective, and simple method of maintaining good pain control.

SPINAL ADMINISTRATION

Since spinal opioid analgesia was introduced in the late 1970s, its use has grown dramatically. It has been utilized in the intraoperative and postoperative settings, for obstetric analgesia, and for chronic pain of malignant and nonmalignant origin (Cousins and Mather 1984). The opioids, generally morphine and related compounds, are given through either epidural or intrathecal routes. Spinal opioids may be given by intermittent injection through reservoir devices or by continuous infusion through implantable and external pumps.

Spinal administration offers potential advantages over the systemic administration of opioids because lower doses produce longer pain relief. For example, 5 mg of morphine given epidurally provides analgesia for 12 to 18 hours. Disadvantages of the spinal route include more difficult drug delivery and a longer onset of action time. Spinal morphine causes satisfactory analgesia after 30 to 60 minutes, compared to 5 to 10 minutes for intravenous morphine (Payne 1987b).

Much has been learned during the last decade about the pharmacology of opioids given by the spinal routes. A sizable proportion of drug injected at the lumbar level intrathecally will ascend in the cerebrospinal fluid (CSF) (fig. 7.2). The same occurs to that fraction of an epidural dose that crosses the dura mater. After intrathecal injection, the less fat-soluble drugs, such as morphine, will remain longer in the CSF and a higher proportion will be free to travel rostrally. With epidural use, drugs of low fat solubility are subject to less vascular absorption and a larger fraction is left to cross the dura. With epidural injections, concentrations of opioids in plasma can be substantial and may contribute to supraspinal analgesia in a fashion similar to that of conventional parenteral injections.

The present evidence suggests that the analgesic action of spinal opioids comes from a direct action with specific receptors in the spinal cord as well as from a supraspinal effect through blood-borne drug. The duration of analgesia is limited by the life span of the occupied opioid receptors at both spinal and cerebral levels. As noted previously, small doses of epidural morphine can produce long periods of analgesia.

It seems that there is a cross-tolerance between systemic and spinally administered opioids and that tolerance to spinal opioids may develop rapidly. Tolerance, in fact, may be a major factor limiting the effectiveness of spinal opioid analgesia.

Indications for the spinal administration of opioids are still being defined. This route may be particularly helpful in patients with severe bilateral or midline opioid-sensitive pain below the level of the umbilicus, who cannot obtain adequate pain relief with systemic opioids because of dose-limiting side effects. Sacral bone metastasis and lumbosacral plexus involvement with tumor, often seen in patients with genitourinary and colon cancers, are a frequent cause of this type of

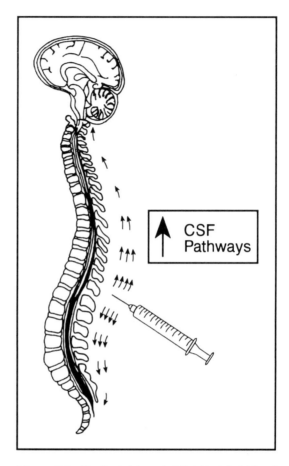

Figure 7.2   The Rostral Ascent of Opioids Administered
by the Spinal Route

pain (Payne 1987b, 1989a). In addition, good results have been reported in patients whose oral intake of morphine was at or below the median four-hour requirement of 20 mg. Poor pain control, however, has
followed spinal opioid use for pain that was poorly sensitive to systemic
opioids (Editorial, Spinal opiates, 1986). Therefore, the spinal administration of opioids may be useful in patients with opioid-sensitive pain
that cannot be managed by conventional routes (table 7.2).

Epidural or intrathecal administration of morphine produces CSF
concentrations one or two times greater than those obtained by the
systemic route and is associated with significant levels of drug in plasma. Thus, blood-borne drug delivery to the brain, combined with rostral CSF redistribution of drug, may cause unwanted supraspinal side

Table 7.2   The Indications for the Spinal Administration of Opioids

Opioid-sensitive pain not managed by conventional routes because of dose-limiting side effects
Severe bilateral or midline pain below the level of the umbilicus
Pelvic pain due to sacral bone metastasis or lumbosacral plexus involvement with tumor

Sources: Editorial, Spinal opiates (1986); Payne (1987b, 1989a).

effects, such as respiratory depression, pruritus, urinary retention, and nausea and vomiting.

The most serious complication of the spinal administration of opioids is respiratory depression, which may occur early (1 to 2 hours) or late (6 to 24 hours). Early respiratory depression is related to systemic absorption of the drug and its supraspinal effect, whereas late respiratory depression is caused by rostral drug flow in the CSF. A 4 to 7 percent incidence of respiratory depression has been reported after intrathecal morphine. However, fatal respiratory depression has not been associated with the chronic use of opioids by the spinal route.

Certain factors that predispose to respiratory depression after the use of spinal opioids have been identified (Payne 1987b, 1989a).

* Advanced age
* The use of large doses of low-fat soluble drugs, such as morphine
* Lack of systemic opioid tolerance
* Marked changes in intrathoracic pressures, such as might occur with end-expiratory ventilation
* The concomitant administration of opioids and other central nervous system depressants by systemic routes

Pruritus occurs in 0 to 80 percent of patients treated with spinal opioids. The characteristics of pruritus are that

* it occurs after acute and chronic administration and is not dose dependent;
* it occurs regardless of the spinal route (i.e., epidural or intrathecal);
* it usually continues for the duration of analgesia;
* it is not segmental, generally occurring on the face and palate;
* it is not related to the preservatives in the drug solution;
* it is not blocked by histamine and may be worsened by coadministration of steroids;
* it occurs more commonly after the administration of systemic or

spinal opioids than after the spinal administration of local anesthetics;

* it may be reversed with naloxone; and
* it may be severe enough to limit therapy.

The mechanism of spinal opioid-induced pruritus is unknown. Urinary retention requiring bladder catheterization is seen in 0.3 to 90 percent of patients treated with spinal opioids. Approximately 70 percent of these cases occurred in elderly men. Urinary retention has been reported with low doses, such as 3 to 4 mg epidural, and can last as long as 18 hours after the administration of spinal opioids. The mechanism of this side effect is unknown, but it may involve a direct effect of opioids on the spinal cord to decrease parasympathetic tone to the bladder.

Nausea and vomiting occur in 15 to 75 percent of postoperative, obstetric, and cancer patients treated with spinal opioids. This complication may occur within 10 to 70 minutes after as little as 1 to 2 mg of intrathecal morphine. However, tolerance to this side effect may develop rapidly.

Minimization of the supraspinal component of the above-noted side effects that are related to rostral CSF redistribution of drug may occur with the use of drugs such as methadone and fentanyl. These drugs are more fat soluble and are rapidly cleared from the CSF before rostral ascent to the brainstem.

Two papers are representative of the medical literature on the use of spinal opioids to control cancer pain not relieved by conventional systemic opioid administration. DuPen et al. (1987) treated 55 cancer patients with metastatic disease and intractable pain; they used an exteriorized epidural catheter for the self-administration of morphine. No catheter infections were found during 3,891 catheter-days of use, and only 18 minor side effects (mostly nausea and vomiting) were noted. No respiratory depression was observed. Hospitalization for pain control was decreased by 90 percent.

Penn and Paice (1987) used intrathecal morphine delivered by implanted continuous infusion or programmable devices to manage 35 cancer patients with uncontrolled pain. Twenty-eight (80 percent) of the patients experienced excellent or good pain relief. Side effects were rare.

Although the use of spinal opioids for pain control represents advancing technology, many questions need to be answered. These scientific questions pertain to optimal drug use (including dosage and pharmacology), understanding and managing tolerance, and the exact role of this treatment modality in clinical practice. A report by Hogan et al.

(1991) placed in perspective the current role of spinal opioids in the management of chronic cancer pain. By aggressively using systemic opioids, they administered epidural morphine to only 15 of 1205 patients (1.2 percent); to achieve successful analgesia, bupivacaine had to be added in half the cases. Complications occurred in 11 of these 16 patients. The investigators concluded that spinal opioids are indicated in only a few selected patients.

Ultimately, because of the invasive nature of drug administration via the spinal route and the associated costs to the patient and family, prospective clinical trials must be performed to compare the effectiveness of spinal opioids to those of current conventional routes.

TRANSDERMAL ADMINISTRATION

The use of the transdermal route for drug delivery is not new. In fact, nitroglycerin, clondine, and scopolamine have been used in this manner. Physiologically, the skin serves as a shield to protect the body from the invasion of microorganisms, viruses, and toxic chemicals and to prevent the loss of important vital materials, such as water, from the body. The skin is relatively impermeable to most substances, with the stratum corneum, a layer of skin, being the principal barrier. This impermeability is more passive than active and is closely connected with a drug's minimal ability to diffuse through the intercellular lipid phase of the stratum corneum.

The Transdermal Therapeutic System (TTS) (ALZA Corporation, Palo Alto, California) is one such transdermal system of drug delivery. The TTS consists of an outer backing membrane in contact with the drug reservoir, a drug reservoir containing the active substance, a microporous membrane of specific permeability, a pressure-sensitive adhesive layer that keeps the system on the skin while offering minimal resistance to drug transport, and a protective film, which the patient removes from the system before application (fig. 7.3). The inclusion of a rate-controlling membrane provides an opportunity to diminish fluctuations in drug levels, thereby reducing the potential for exposure to subtherapeutic or toxic serum concentrations.

The TTS was originally developed to test the use of transdermal scopolamine to prevent or relieve travel sickness and nausea. Scopolamine had long been known to be active against this problem but, because of its marked side effects, had been used infrequently in conventional dosage forms. Clinical studies with TTS (scopolamine) for motion sickness demonstrated that the release of scopolamine from the system had the desired therapeutic effect without eliciting the bothersome side effects associated with the other forms of dosage.

Figure 7.3   A Transdermal Therapeutic System for the Release of Fentanyl

Shortly after the application of TTS, the drug (scopolamine) is released. It saturates the binding sites in the skin. Thereafter, a continuous controlled release of the drug occurs for up to 72 hours. Scopolamine travels via the circulatory system to the target site. After the system is removed from the skin, the drug concentration in the systemic circulation falls to an ineffective level (Heilmann 1978).

Advantages of transdermal drug administration include a high degree of patient acceptability of the noninvasive technique; reduced variations in serum concentrations of the drug, leading to improvement in response and minimization of adverse effects; improved patient compliance as a result of longer dosing intervals and less frequent administration; elimination of gastrointestinal absorption problems related to oral dosing; reduction of drug metabolism because the liver is initially bypassed; and the use of drugs with short biologic half-lives.

Fentanyl citrate is a synthetic opioid analgesic, approximately 75 times more potent than morphine, which is used primarily for sedation in the perioperative setting or for analgesia during dental surgery. Physicochemical characteristics of fentanyl, such as high potency, skin compatibility, low molecular weight, and appropriate solubility, make it suitable for rate-controlled transdermal delivery. Fentanyl is eliminated from the body predominantly by biotransformation in the liver. Studies of fentanyl given by continuous intravenous infusion for postoperative analgesia suggest that the dosage of approximately 100 μg/hour is effective and well tolerated in adults (Plezia et al. 1989).

Two studies (Plezia et al. 1989; Caplan et al. 1989) evaluated TTS (fentanyl) in the postoperative setting. Plezia et al. (1989) studied eight patients, who had undergone orthopedic surgery, for 24 hours postoperatively. Two hours before surgery, the TTS (fentanyl) was applied to each patient's upper anterior chest wall, and it remained in place for 24 hours. The nominal delivery rate of the system was 75 μg/hour. Serum samples were obtained over a 72-hour period for pharmacokinetic study in five patients. Transdermal administration of fentanyl was very well tolerated in this group of patients. Adverse reactions were minimal. Pharmacokinetic analysis suggested continuous delivery of the drug after a two-hour lag period, with prolonged elimination. Prolongation of fentanyl elimination resulted from the formation of a deposit of the drug in the fatty skin tissue underneath the transdermal system. After removal of the device, drug diffused away from the site at a gradually declining rate, giving the appearance of prolonged elimination. This phenomenon was responsible for the lag time from the application of the transdermal system to the appearance of drug in circulation. In that setting, the transdermal administration of fentanyl seemed to be a viable alternative to conventional routes of opioid administration and warranted further investigation.

In a larger, double-blind, placebo-controlled study, Caplan et al. (1989) evaluated the safety and efficacy of transdermal fentanyl for postoperative pain management in 42 healthy adult patients undergoing major shoulder surgery. The TTS (fentanyl) was used, and, as in the previous study, fentanyl was delivered at a rate of 75 μg/hour. TTS (fentanyl) was applied to the skin immediately before surgery and was worn for 24 hours. Patients in the fentanyl group required significantly less morphine than did the placebo group during the 24-hour period that the systems were in place and during the first 12 hours after removal. The incidence of vomiting and lowered respiratory rate, however, was higher. As noted by the authors, the slow decline in serum fentanyl levels may offer a potential advantage in that the transition to other forms of pain management may occur without an abrupt loss of analgesia. The investigators concluded that transdermal fentanyl seems to be safe and effective after orthopedic surgery in healthy adult patients and that the transdermal delivery of fentanyl produces an agreeable, constant quality of pain control that is superior to conventional therapy with intramuscular morphine.

In 1989, Miser et al. reported their experience in using TTS delivery to treat five cancer patients with transdermal fentanyl. Patients were initially begun on a continuous intravenous infusion of fentanyl to achieve satisfactory pain control. After this endpoint was reached, TTS (fentanyl) patches were applied to the chest wall, back, or upper arm and were routinely changed every 24 hours, as preclinical testing with these systems had demonstrated constant drug delivery for this period. Also, skin sites were rotated with each application. The TTS delivered drug at 25, 50, or 100 μg/hour. The five patients, who were 16 to 68 years old, had a history of poor pain control due to an inability to take oral analgesics or because these drugs were ineffective in controlling pain. Overall, the patients experienced satisfactory pain relief for periods of 3 to 156 days (mean, 145 days) using continuous transdermal delivery of fentanyl. Dosages were adjusted to each patient's need and varied from 75 to 350 μg/hour, with a median of 225 μg/hour. No patient developed skin irritation at the site of application. Major clinical difficulties noted in the study included the delay in obtaining steady-state serum concentrations of fentanyl (which led to minor overdosing in two patients) and the prolonged period of continued fentanyl effect after TTS removal. This prolonged effect became an important clinical issue when unrelated medical complications arose suddenly in patients and a more rapid change in opioid level was desired. As noted by the authors, transdermal delivery of opioid provides an ideal analgesic modality for patients with chronic pain who are in stable clinical condition and who otherwise would have required parenteral opioids. In this study, transdermal fentanyl permitted home care for three of the five patients.

In a larger study, Simmonds et al. (1989) investigated TTS (fentanyl) in 39 patients with various forms of advanced cancer. The opioid treatment was converted to oral morphine and titrated to a stable dose. Conversion was made to TTS, which was applied every three days. Immediate-release morphine was prescribed for breakthrough pain. There were 16 female and 23 male patients, with a median age of 61 years. The median morphine stabilization dosage was 120 mg/day. The median dosage of fentanyl at the start of the study was 50 μg/hour (range, 25 to 225) and the median current or final dosage was 100 μg/hour (range, 25 to 525). More than half of the patients increased their dosage by 50 percent or more while on the study. The patients were able to maintain the TTS patch through a variety of concomitant events, such as surgery for pathologic fracture, herpes zoster infection, and chemotherapy infusions. Thus, the authors suggested, the clinical use and safety of TTS (fentanyl) in this group of cancer patients have been demonstrated. Patient compliance and acceptance were excellent.

Payne (1992) provided guidelines for the use of transdermal fentanyl.

- Patients with stable baseline pain and minimal incident pain are good candidates for this route of administration because frequent dose adjustments are difficult to achieve with transdermal fentanyl. It is usually necessary to obtain adequate baseline pain control with conventional opioid dosing before initiating transdermal fentanyl treatment.
- Because of the unique pharmacokinetics of fentanyl delivered transdermally, the liberal use of immediate-release analgesics for rescue dosing is often necessary, especially when therapy is being started or when the dosage is being adjusted. The average 72-hour

rescue dose of analgesics is used to calculate dose changes of transdermal fentanyl at the time of the next patch application.

• Rotate skin sites to minimize variations in blood level due to the excess accumulation of subcutaneous deposits of fentanyl. Warn patients about poor skin adhesion resulting from sweating and hair growth.

• Because of the increased risks of side effects associated with the use of long-acting opioids, transdermal fentanyl should not be routinely administered with controlled-release morphine, methadone, or levorphanol.

To aid in the calculation of the dosage of transdermal fentanyl, Johanson (1992) recommended the following approximate equivalencies in the chronic, steady state:

25-μg/hour patch = 10 mg oral morphine every four hours
50-μg/hour patch = 20 mg oral morphine every four hours
75-μg/hour patch = 30 mg oral morphine every four hours
100-μg/hour patch = 40 mg oral morphine every four hours

The success of the TTS (fentanyl) model is directly related to the permeability of fentanyl across the skin barrier. The same is not true for morphine. Utilizing an animal model, Sugibayashi, Sakanoue, and Morimoto (1989) studied the role of skin penetration enhancers added to morphine hydrochloride. They found that the addition of azone and N-methyl-2 pyrrolidone to a morphine solution significantly enhanced the skin permeation of morphine. Much more preclinical research is needed in this area before topical morphine can be clinically tested in patients.

Summary

Oral morphine is the drug of choice for chronic severe pain. In most cases, it can be given by this route until death. Administered as an immediate-release preparation at four-hour intervals, oral morphine produces analgesia within 60 minutes, with a peak effect at 1.5 to 2.0 hours and a four- to seven-hour duration. Because of wide individual variation in the metabolism of morphine, there is a broad therapeutic dose range for good pain control. The oral : parenteral potency in chronic pain is 2–3:1; thus, the usual starting dose in an opioid-naive patient is 20 to 30 mg every four hours. Based on pharmacokinetic studies, older patients require smaller doses of morphine for pain control than do younger patients. Use four-hour dosing of oral morphine for initial pain stabilization and for breakthrough pain when long-acting preparations are employed.

As evidenced by a study from the United Kingdom (White et al. 1991), there is considerable confusion and misperception concerning the use of controlled-release morphine such as MS Contin. This, in turn, has led to its misuse, especially in regard to the frequency of administration and escalation of the dosage. Multiple clinical studies have demonstrated that controlled-release morphine administered at 12-hour intervals produces pain control equivalent to that of oral morphine given every 4 hours. Controlled-release oral morphine should be used for maintenance therapy once the patient's morphine requirement is determined; it is inappropriate for use "as needed." When converting patients from immediate-release oral morphine preparations to the controlled-release formulation, use a potency ratio of 1 : 1.

Continuous parenteral infusions of opioids, regardless of the route, are safe and are associated with low toxicity except in those rare patients requiring more than 4 grams of intravenous morphine per day in whom seizures may occur because of the excess accumulation of bisulfite preservatives. The continuous subcutaneous route offers better quality-of-life satisfaction for the patient than does the intravenous route.

Continuous parenteral infusions of opioids coupled with patient-controlled analgesia bolus for breakthrough pain is highly effective for relieving pain and can be safely administered at home. The PCA technique is most advantageous in managing incident pain.

Utilizing a mucosal membrane route (such as sublingual, buccal, or rectal) to administer opioid analgesics produces a more rapid onset and a longer duration of analgesia. This route is especially useful when the patient is near death and unable to swallow.

Giving opioids via the spinal route is another alternative in providing analgesia. Lower dosages of spinal morphine administered either intrathecally or epidurally produce longer analgesia than do those delivered by conventional routes. Indications for the spinal administration of opioids are still being defined. Many scientific questions regarding the use of spinal opioids to manage chronic cancer pain remain unanswered, including optimal drug use, tolerance, and the exact role of this treatment modality in clinical practice. Until these answers are provided, conventional routes of administering opioids remain the standard of care except in selected patients.

Technology is available to deliver drugs transdermally in a rate-controlled fashion over a long period. Fentanyl, a synthetic opioid analgesic, is 75 times more potent than morphine and can penetrate the skin. Like the controlled-release preparations of morphine, transdermal fentanyl is useful in patients with stable chronic pain and minimal discomfort associated with movement.

Chapter 8

Adjuvant Analgesic Drugs

The use of drugs added to opioid analgesics to improve the control of cancer pain is unclear at best. Even the terminology is confusing: some authors refer to these agents as *coanalgesics* (Twycross and Hanks 1984), whereas others call them *adjuvant analgesic drugs* (Foley and Arbit 1989; Payne 1991). There also seems to be little agreement as to what agents to include in this category. To ensure a uniform approach, I shall use the term *adjuvant analgesic drugs*, and I include in this group anticonvulsants, phenothiazines, antidepressants, antihistamines, steroids, and antibiotics.

Anticonvulsants

Anticonvulsants, such as phenytoin and carbamazepine, are well-known effective drugs for the management of pain in chronic neuralgias (such as trigeminal neuralgia, postherpetic neuralgia, glossopharyngeal neuralgia, and posttraumatic neuralgias). In cancer pain, carbamazepine is useful in managing the acute, shocklike neuralgic pain in the cranial and cervical distribution caused by infiltration by the tumor or surgical injury to the nerve. It also is effective in patients with involvement of the lumbosacral plexus (Payne 1991).

Phenothiazines

The phenothiazines, with the possible exception of methotrimeprazine, play a minimal role in the management of cancer pain. Methotrimeprazine, available only in the parenteral form, exhibits analgesic properties and is useful in special circumstances, such as opioid tolerance or the need to avoid the constipating effects of opioids while maintaining analgesia. The combination of fluphenazine and a tricyclic antidepressant may prove useful for the management of nerve injury pain (Payne 1991), but, as in other areas, agreement is not uniform (Hanks 1984). Combining a phenothiazine, such as prochlorperazine, and an opioid analgesic heightens only sedation and not pain control. Because of this and other enhancements of side effects, the routine use of a phenothiazine as an antiemetic combined with an opioid is strongly condemned.

Antidepressants

Tricyclic antidepressants are one group of drugs that most agree play a role in pain management. Their direct analgesic effects are provided by blockage of the reuptake of serotonin and norepinephrine at the central nervous system synapses. Another mechanism of action may relate to the emotional component of pain perception. In a review, Magni, Conlon, and Arsie (1987) concluded that the tricyclic antidepressants seem to be useful in reducing cancer pain that may or may not be associated with depressive symptoms. The dosage is similar to that used in the treatment of depression. Furthermore, the authors suggested that, when the tricyclic antidepressants are used concurrently with opioids, a dose reduction in the opioid analgesics and a potentiation of analgesia are possible. Others (Foley and Arbit 1989; Payne 1991) thought that analgesic effects are evident at lower doses (e.g., 10 to 150 mg daily for amitriptyline) than are the antidepressant effects. In one of the few controlled clinical trials, amitriptyline demonstrated significant analgesia in the management of postherpetic neuralgia as compared to placebo (Watson et al. 1982).

Antihistamines

Of the antihistamines, hydroxyzine is the most frequently utilized in clinical practice. It may produce additive analgesia, in doses of 25 to 100 mg daily, when combined with opioids (Payne 1991).

Steroids

Steroids are another group of drug that may act as adjuvant analgesic agents in certain clinical circumstances, such as spinal cord compression due to tumor, brain metastases, and compression or infiltration of nerve by tumor. In these instances, steroids offer pain relief by decreasing the soft tissue swelling in the area of the tumor focus. Dexamethasone seems to be the steroid of choice for these clinical situations (Twycross and Hanks 1984). Claims for the use of steroids, for example, in patients with soft tissue tumor infiltration and hepatomegaly (Hanks and Justins 1992) are poorly substantiated.

Antibiotics

Antibiotics may be useful in certain clinical circumstances, such as acute infection associated with malignant ulceration (Bruera and MacDonald 1986) and cellulitis (Hanks and Justins 1992). Bruera and MacDonald (1986) observed seven patients with locally advanced head and neck carcinoma who had a sudden increase in their pain that improved with antibiotics. All of these patients had large ulcerated masses surrounded by chronic swelling and erythema before the onset of the severe pain. Significant relief from pain was obtained in all patients within three days of starting the antibiotic therapy. The authors suggested that acute local infection is probably a frequent event and should be suspected in patients with head and neck cancers who show a rapidly changing pattern of pain. Furthermore, signs of local infection as well as fever and leukocytosis may be absent, and a therapeutic trial of antibiotics may be necessary in these cases.

Amphetamines

There is a resurgence of interest in the use of amphetamines as adjuvant analgesic agents in the management of chronic cancer pain. In 1977 Forrest et al. were the first to demonstrate that dextroamphetamine enhanced the analgesic effect of morphine in 450 patients with acute postoperative pain. The investigators found, in this double-blind, single-dose study, that analgesia was augmented with the combination of drugs. Dextroamphetamine, 5 mg, in conjunction with a certain dose of morphine provided relief of pain equivalent to that obtained with one and one-half times that dose of morphine taken alone. Adding dextroamphetamine, 10 mg, to morphine has the analgesic effect of approximately twice that dose of morphine alone. The Forrest et al. (1977) study, however, was in the acute pain noncancer setting.

In 1982, Joshi et al. (1982) reported their experience with amphetamines in terminally ill cancer patients. Nineteen patients were given dextroamphetamine at a starting dosage of 2.5 mg every six hours. In this noncontrolled study, 16 patients were evaluable for response. Improvements, as recorded by two physician observers, were noted in mood (87 percent), activity level (75 percent), pain (70 percent), and appetite (43 percent). In a subsequent controlled clinical study with a double-blind, cross-over design, Bruera, Carraro, et al. (1986) compared a mild amphetamine, mazindol, with a placebo to determine its effectiveness for symptom control in 30 terminally ill cancer patients. The authors reported that mazindol was associated with severe toxicity in the form of delirium (2 patients) that required the discontinuation of the treatment. The use of mazindol, as employed in this study, did not significantly improve comfort in any of the patients. However, the data suggested that the use of mazindol decreased the intensity of the pain and the consumption of oral analgesics. Patients enrolled in this study had only mild or moderate pain.

In 1987, this same group (Bruera, Chadwick, Brenneis, et al. 1987) evaluated the adjuvant analgesic properties of methylphenidate in 32 patients with advanced cancer. All patients were receiving opioids on a regular basis and were treated with methylphenidate (10 mg orally with breakfast and 5 mg orally with lunch) for three days versus placebo in a randomized double-blind, cross-over study. In the 28 evaluable patients, methylphenidate potentiated the analgesic effects of the opioids, decreased drowsiness, and significantly increased the level of patient activity. After the study was completed, the investigator and the patient chose methylphenidate blindly as a more useful drug in 23 cases (82 percent) and 20 cases (71 percent), respectively. Severe toxicity was not observed. Although low-dose methylphenidate combined with opioid analgesics may have a role in managing severe cancer pain, the authors cautioned that amphetamines may enhance mental abnormalities in this situation. Therefore, until future study, Bruera, Chadwick, Brenneis, et al. (1987) did not recommend the more general use of methylphenidate for improving the comfort of terminally ill patients.

Butyrophenones

The butyrophenone haloperidol potentiates morphine analgesia in animals; however, there are few clinical data to support these effects in humans. In a review of the literature, Hanks (1984) was unable to substantiate an opioid-sparing effect of haloperidol and did not advocate its use.

Finally, several groups of drug should be avoided in the management of chronic cancer pain: the benzodiazepines, sedative-hypnotics such as the barbiturates, canabinoids, and cocaine (Payne 1991).

Summary

Despite confusion regarding the terminology, adjuvant analgesics play an important role in the management of pain. The anticonvulsants, especially carbamazepine, are helpful in managing neuropathic pain, as are the tricyclic antidepressants, such as amitriptyline. The routine use of a phenothiazine as an antiemetic enhances only sedation and not pain control and therefore is inappropriate. Steroids, mainly dexamethasone, are indicated in cases of the involvement or compression of the nervous system by tumor. Antibiotics may improve pain control in patients with acute local infections, as occurs in patients with advanced head and neck cancer. Despite encouraging preliminary results, the routine use of amphetamines as adjuvant therapy is not recommended.

Chapter 9

Complications of Pharmacologic Therapy

Although chronic pain may be effectively controlled with a wide variety of pharmacologic agents, this is often associated with untoward side effects. In some cases, these side effects become so burdensome that they interfere with the goal of patient comfort. Therefore, an appreciation of the side effects of pharmacologic pain control and how they are managed is critical to good patient care.

Opioids

Certain risks expose the patient to a greater likelihood of having a drug-related complication. Age is a major factor. Older patients are more sensitive to opioids and their side effects than are younger patients. Prior treatment with opioids and the route of administration are also important. For example, sublingual, buccal, and rectal administration of morphine has fewer side effects than does the oral route. The presence of underlying medical problems, especially pulmonary disease, may enhance untoward reactions to pain management therapies. Patients with pulmonary dysfunction are at greater risk for developing opioid-induced respiratory depression than are patients with normal lung function.

In 1987, Ventafridda et al. (1987) reported their two-year experience using the World Health Organization three-step treatment for cancer pain. In brief, this analgesia ladder starts with nonopioids, such as aspirin, acetaminophen, and other nonsteroidal anti-inflammatory drugs. As the pain progresses, the next step is the use of weak opioids (codeine, for example). The final step, if the pain persists, is the utilization of the strong opioids (i.e., morphine and related compounds). Adjuvant analgesics may be used as well.

The investigators calculated the percentage of days on which side effects were present during a two-month follow-up of patients treated.

Over the entire span of the three-step treatment, the most frequent side effects were dry mouth, drowsiness, constipation, sweating, and nausea/vomiting (table 9.1).

Not surprisingly, there were no side effects in more patients given nonopioids than in those given strong opioids (39 percent versus 21 percent). More dry mouth, drowsiness, constipation, and sweating were reported by the patients treated with the strong opioids, predominantly morphine, than by the patients given either nonopioids or weak opioids.

DRY MOUTH

Although the study by Ventafridda et al. (1987) identified dry mouth as the most frequent side effect of treatment using the WHO analgesia ladder, it is difficult to attribute this complication to a single drug because most patients were taking multiple drugs. Therefore, a study by White et al. (1989) is helpful in identifying a cause for this complication. These investigators studied the prevalence of dryness of the mouth in patients with cancer to determine if it was related to the use of morphine. All patients admitted to the Continuing Care Unit, Royal Marsden Hospital, during an eight-week period were entered into the study except those who had other reasons for having a dry mouth (such as those receiving radiation therapy, surgery, chemotherapy, or the like). Data were obtained from 199 patients. One hundred thirty-one patients were using opioid analgesics, and 67 were taking morphine. One hundred nineteen of 199 patients (57 percent)

Table 9.1   The Frequency of Side Effects Associated with the WHO Analgesia Ladder

Side Effect	Frequency
Dry mouth	39%
Drowsiness	38%
Constipation	35%
Sweating	23%
Nausea/vomiting	22%
Stomach ache	17%
Agitation	16%
Itching	10%
Blood loss	6%
None	24%

Source: Ventafridda et al. (1987).

reported dryness of the mouth at some time during the course of treatment; of these 119, 42 (37 percent) had a dry mouth most or all of the time. There was no significant correlation between the severity of the mouth dryness and sex, age, primary diagnosis, reason for admission, the wearing of dentures, oral candidiasis, or smoking. Analysis showed a highly significant association between the use of morphine and dryness of the mouth. When the results were controlled for concurrent treatment, patients receiving morphine were approximately four times more likely to have dry mouth of any severity than were patients taking weak opioids, nonopioids, or no analgesics.

The mechanisms for the adverse effect of morphine were unclear. As noted by the authors, recognition of this side effect is important, and careful attention should be paid to oral comfort and hygiene.

RESPIRATORY DEPRESSION

In a review of analgesic drug therapy for chronic cancer pain, Foley and Inturrisi (1987) suggested that the most common side effects of opioid analgesics are sedation, nausea and vomiting, constipation, and respiratory depression. With the exception of respiratory depression, these are similar to those reported by Ventafridda et al. (1987) (table 9.2).

Respiratory depression is potentially the most serious side effect of opioid therapy. Morphine and related drugs act on brainstem respiratory centers to produce dose-dependent respiratory depression. Therapeutic doses of morphine may depress all phases of respiration. However, as carbon dioxide accumulates, it stimulates the respiratory centers, resulting in a compensatory increase in respiratory rate, which, in turn, hides the degree of respiratory depression. At equivalent doses,

Table 9.2 The Clinically Important Side Effects of Opioids

CNS-related Side Effects	Non-CNS-related Side Effects
Drowsiness/sedation	Dry mouth
Nausea/vomiting	Constipation
Agitation, nightmares, anxiety, euphoria, dysphoria, depression, paranoia, hallucinations	Sweating
	Itching
	Urinary retention
Respiratory depression	

Sources: Foley and Inturrisi (1987); *Medical Letter* (1989a); Ventafridda et al. (1987).

Note: Side effects are listed in decreasing order of frequency. CNS, central nervous system.

all morphine-related drugs produce the same degree of respiratory depression. For these reasons, Foley and Inturrisi (1987) suggested that patients with impaired respiratory function or bronchial asthma are at greater risk for experiencing clinically significant respiratory depression in response to the usual dosages of these drugs.

Respiratory depression usually occurs with the acute administration of morphine to an opioid-naive patient and is often accompanied by other signs of central nervous system depression, such as sedation and confusion. A tolerance of the effect develops rapidly with repeated administration of the drug, thus typically allowing opioid analgesics to be used in the management of chronic pain without significant risk of respiratory depression.

If respiratory depression occurs, it may be reversed by the administration of the specific opioid antagonist naloxone. In patients being treated with opioids chronically who develop respiratory depression, naloxone diluted 1:10 should be titrated carefully to prevent the precipitation of severe withdrawal symptoms (Foley and Inturrisi 1987).

The major effect of the opioids on the central nervous system is sedation or drowsiness. Because of an additive effect, clinicians must exercise care in the use of other CNS depressants, such as alcohol, barbiturates, and benzodiazepines in combination with opioids. A tolerance of sedation usually develops within the first several days of the chronic administration of opioids.

NAUSEA AND VOMITING

Opioid analgesics produce nausea and vomiting by acting on the medullary chemoreceptor trigger zone. The tendency of these drugs to cause nausea and vomiting varies from patient to patient, so there may be some advantage to changing opioids in patients experiencing this side effect. Alternatively, antiemetics may be combined with the opioid. However, the choice of antiemetics is important because drugs, such as the phenothiazines, may only enhance opioid-induced sedation.

OTHER SIDE EFFECTS ON THE CENTRAL NERVOUS SYSTEM

Other, less frequent side effects on the CNS include nightmares, anxiety, agitation, euphoria, dysphoria, depression, paranoia, and hallucinations. These generally occur with high doses of opioids, with the possible exception of meperidine and methadone (*Medical Letter* 1989a). Accumulation of the metabolite normeperidine in patients treated chronically with meperidine causes excitation of the CNS. For this reason, this drug is not recommended for use in the management of chronic cancer pain. Clinicians must also take care when using methadone. Because of its long half-life (15 to 30 hours), methadone in chronic dosing can lead to drug accumulation, which can lead to oversedation and, rarely, coma.

CONSTIPATION

Constipation is a common side effect of opioid analgesics. These drugs act at multiple sites throughout the gastrointestinal tract and spinal cord to cause a decrease in intestinal secretions and peristalsis. The net effect is constipation. A tolerance of the smooth muscle effects of opioids develops very slowly, so constipation persists when these drugs are used for chronic pain. When opioids are started, give careful attention to managing this side effect. Measures such as increasing ambulation and fluid intake, beginning a diet high in fiber, or trying a bulk laxative should be initiated. The daily administration of a stool softener is also helpful.

THE RETENTION OF URINE

Another side effect of the opioid analgesics is bladder spasm and an increase in smooth muscle sphincter tone leading to urinary retention. This is most common in older patients and is transient. The itching and sweating associated with opioids is most likely related to histamine release.

ADDICTION

Fear of addiction to opioid analgesics remains a major impediment to good pain control. This perception is shared by both the patient and caregivers and is further reinforced by the ongoing battle with illicit drug use as highlighted in the news media. Physicians are often reluctant to prescribe opioids until "the last" because of this problem. A recent survey of 200 Wisconsin physicians by Weissman, Joranson, and Hopwood (1991) found that physicians were less concerned about regulatory drug use investigation than about addiction, tolerance, or respiratory depression.

In a similar fashion, patients are afraid to start treatment with the opioids, often despite the presence of severe uncontrolled pain, because they do not want to be "hooked" on these drugs. Many times the patient's negative perception of opioids is strongly reinforced by family members.

Much of the confusion regarding opioids and addiction is related to a poor understanding of terminology, specifically, *tolerance, physical dependence*, and *psychologic dependence* or *addiction*. *Tolerance* occurs when, after repeated administrations of a drug, a larger dose must be given to obtain the effects observed with the original dose. On the other hand, *physical dependence* refers to an altered physiologic state produced by the repeated administration of a drug to the extent that a sudden cessation of the drug results in withdrawal symptoms. Finally, *psychologic dependence* or *addiction* is a behavioral pattern of drug use characterized by overwhelming involvement with the use of the drug and the securing of its supply and a high tendency to relapse after withdrawal (Jaffe 1985).

Tolerance. Tolerance, or the need for escalating opioid doses to maintain adequate analgesia, seems to develop in all patients receiving opioids chronically. The rate of development of this phenomenon, however, varies greatly among cancer patients. Data from animals show that tolerance to morphine occurs in rodents within 24 hours, reaching a maximum within one week. This suggests that more than one week of patient exposure to this drug may lead to tolerance (Chapman and Hill 1989).

The first indication of tolerance is the patient's complaint that the duration of analgesia is decreased from that of the initial administration. Frequently, the patient is labeled as a "clock watcher," a sign that is often viewed by caregivers as an early sign of addiction.

Studies indicate that there are three patterns of drug use in cancer patients:

- rapidly escalating dosages of opioids associated with increasing pain and/or anxiety,
- stable dosages of opioids for long periods (weeks to months) without escalation or reduction of the dosage, and
- discontinuance of opioid drugs with effective analgesia from cancer therapies or anesthetic or neurosurgical approaches.

These patterns are independent of the route of administering the drug, with progression of painful disease as the overriding factor determining the escalation of the dosage. Although the rate of developing tolerance may vary from patient to patient, a sudden dramatic increase in opioid requirements may well signal a progression of the cancer rather than the development of tolerance.

There seems to be no limit to tolerance. Regardless of the current dosage, dose escalation is appropriate when the goal is effective analgesia. The majority of patients treated by the Supportive Care Program at Memorial Sloan-Kettering Cancer Center required doses in the range of 5 to 300 mg of intramuscular morphine equivalents daily. Some patients required very high doses (Foley 1989). Inexperienced physicians may misinterpret these high doses as inappropriate. They undermedicate patients because of their concern for using only standard dosages rather than seeking adequate analgesia as the endpoint.

Of equal importance is the recognition that cross-tolerance is incomplete. Changing patients from one opioid analgesic to another can improve analgesia.

Finally, tolerance of the various side effects of opioids occurs at different rates. Tolerance of respiratory depression develops rapidly, whereas tolerance of constipation develops very slowly. The rapid development of tolerance of the respiratory depressant effects of opioids allows the escalation of dosages in some patients to very high levels.

Physical Dependence. Physical dependence is the pharmacologic effect of opioids. Withdrawal symptoms occur when the drug is stopped. The severity of withdrawal is a function of the duration and dosage of opioid that was discontinued. Patients treated with therapeutic doses of morphine several times a day for one to two weeks will have only mild symptoms that may not be recognized as withdrawal when the drug is stopped. These symptoms may be even less pronounced when the opioid is one that is slowly eliminated, such as methadone (Jaffe 1985).

The onset of withdrawal is heralded by the patient's report of feelings of anxiety, nervousness, irritability, and alternating chills and hot flushes. A prominent withdrawal sign is wetness, including salivation, lacrimation, rhinorrhea, and diaphoresis. Nausea and vomiting, abdominal cramps, insomnia, and, rarely, multifocal myoclonus may occur at the peak intensity of the withdrawal syndrome. The timing of withdrawal is a function of the elimination half-life of the opioid to which the patient has become physically dependent. For example, symptoms will appear within 6 to 12 hours and reach a peak at 24 to 72 hours after the cessation of a short half-life drug such as morphine. With methadone, which has a long half-life, withdrawal symptoms may be delayed for 36 to 48 hours. Even in patients in whom pain has been completely relieved by a therapeutic procedure, it is necessary to decrease the opioid dosage slowly to prevent withdrawal symptoms.

The usual daily dose required to prevent withdrawal is equal to one-fourth of the previous daily dose, and it is administered every six hours, or four times per day. This initial withdrawal regimen is administered for two days and then reduced by one-half. This amount is also divided into doses given four times daily for two days. After two days on this dose, the patient can stop the opioid. Thus, a patient who had been receiving 240 mg of morphine per day for pain control would require an initial dose of 60 mg administered in 15 mg doses every six hours (Foley and Inturrisi 1987).

The administration of an opioid antagonist, such as naloxone, to a physically dependent patient immediately precipitates the withdrawal syndrome. Patients being treated with repeated doses of a morphinelike agonist to the point where they are physically dependent may experience an opioid withdrawal reaction when given a mixed agonist-antagonist, like pentazocine. Prior exposure to a morphinelike drug greatly increases a patient's sensitivity to the antagonist component of a mixed agonist-antagonist drug.

Psychologic Dependence.   Tolerance and physical dependence are predictable pharmacologic effects seen in response to the repeated administration of opioids in both humans and laboratory animals. These effects are distinctly different from the abnormal behavioral patterns seen in some individuals and described by the term *psychologic dependence* or *addiction.* Addiction is characterized by a continued craving for opioids as manifested by compulsive drug-seeking behavior and overwhelming involvement in the procurement and use of the drug. The development of addiction is a complex phenomenon in which the type of individual, the reason for drug use, the environment, and the drug play major and, at times, equivalent roles. This concept was well described in the epidemic addiction seen in Vietnam War veterans who rapidly discontinued their heroin use once home, without the use of maintenance programs and with low rates of relapse (Foley 1989).

It is clearly possible for patients taking opioids on a chronic basis, such as those with cancer pain, to be physically dependent without evidence of addiction. As noted by Angell (1982), addiction among patients who receive opioids for pain is exceedingly unlikely, and the incidence is probably no greater than 0.1 percent. Further support for this low addiction rate comes from a study by Chapman and Hill (1989). These investigators studied 26 patients who required opioid analgesics for severe oral mucositis after bone marrow transplantation. Twelve patients self-administered morphine via a patient-controlled analgesia system for two weeks. The other fourteen patients acted as controls and were given morphine by routine staff-controlled continuous infusion procedures. Self-administering patients used significantly less morphine than did the controls and still achieved the same amount of pain control. In addition, the self-administering patients terminated drug use sooner than did the control patients. The investigators concluded that the results support the assumption that self-administration of opioids in a medical setting does not put patients at risk for overmedication or addiction.

As reported by Hoffman et al. (1991), a special problem is pain management in cancer patients who are abusing opioids before the onset of the cancer. These investigators described the difficulty in pain management due to problems of distinguishing tolerance from disease progression, concurrent methadone maintenance, and drug-seeking behavior. Suggested guidelines for the management of this problem are to

- provide early psychologic help;
- take complaints of pain at face value and investigate them as necessary
- set limits (e.g., through a medication contract), which is of critical importance;
- prescribe medication on a time-contingent basis; and
- continue the maintenance dose of patients on methadone maintenance while their pain is being treated with other opioid agonists.

Nonsteroidal Anti-inflammatory Drugs

The nonsteroidal anti-inflammatory drugs are often used in the management of chronic pain. Indeed, this group of drugs comprises the first step of the WHO analgesia ladder. Acetaminophen has minimal anti-inflammatory effect and lacks the side effect profile of the NSAIDs. Chronic high dosing can produce renal damage. Salicylates, such as aspirin, in high doses cause gastric irritation, which often limits their use clinically. Also, aspirin at any dose interferes with platelet function, which can lead to bleeding problems.

As a group, the NSAIDs produce similar adverse effects, but the frequency and severity vary with the individual and the specific drug. The major toxicities of the NSAIDs are gastrointestinal, hematologic, renal, and central nervous system (table 9.3).

All NSAIDs can cause dyspepsia and untoward gastrointestinal effects, including bleeding, ulceration, and perforation in patients treated chronically with these drugs. They interfere with platelet function and can cause bleeding. NSAIDs decrease renal blood flow, cause fluid retention, and may cause renal failure in some patients, especially elderly people. All NSAIDs can cause dizziness, anxiety, drowsiness,

Table 9.3   The Clinically Important
Side Effects of Nonsteroidal
Anti-inflammatory Drugs

Gastrointestinal irritation and ulceration
Bleeding due to platelet dysfunction
Impaired renal function
CNS[a] toxicity, including dizziness, anxiety,
    drowsiness, tinnitus, and confusion

Sources: Enck (1991); *Medical Letter* (1989b).
[a]CNS, central nervous system.

tinnitus, and confusion, which may occur initially and disappear with further use. Other less common side effects, such as hepatitis, pancreatitis, and the like, have also been noted (*Medical Letter* 1989b).

Summary

To prevent the development of drug-induced side effects, physicians must recognize and address factors such as age, impaired pulmonary function, and the like during therapy for pain management. A minority of patients treated by the WHO analgesia ladder experience no side effects. Strong opioids (namely, morphine) produce more side effects than do either nonopioids or weak opioids. Finally, NSAIDs are frequently used in managing pain, but their role is often limited by side effects, especially gastrointestinal distress.

Tolerance seems to develop in all patients receiving opioids on a chronic basis and may occur after a week or more of morphine therapy. It is important to understand physical dependence because of the occurrence of withdrawal symptoms, which may be subtle or significant, depending on the duration and dosage of opioids being used when these drugs are stopped. Clinically, this problem can be avoided by a gradual decrease in the daily dosages of opioids. The incidence of addiction in cancer patients taking opioids chronically is probably no greater than 0.1 percent and is not a valid reason for physicians to undertreat patients with severe pain.

Chapter 10

Bone Pain

Bone pain due to cancer metastasis is common. The most frequent primary sites leading to bone metastases are the breast, lung, and prostate. Autopsy studies have identified bone metastases in up to 85 percent of patients dying of these cancers. Most other primary tumors can spread to bone, including renal, thyroid, endometrial, cervical, bladder, and gastrointestinal tract cancers, but these sites account for less than 20 percent of patients with bone metastases. Although the presence of metastatic bone disease generally denotes a poor prognosis, a sizable proportion of patients will live for several months to years. For example, the median survival for metastatic breast cancer is one to two years but, for subgroups of patients with bone metastasis only, a median survival of four years has been reported. The median survival in patients with metastatic prostate cancer is two years, but individual survival varies widely. In contrast, almost all patients with bone metastasis from lung cancer die within one year.

Pain, pathologic fractures, hypercalcemia, neurologic impairment, and immobility are the complications of bone metastases which adversely affect the quality of life for these patients. Neurologic deficits in the form of cranial nerve paralysis and headache are often seen in patients with tumor metastasis at the base of the skull. Involvement of the vertebral body and sacral bone may present diagnostic problems because metastases in these locations may cause not local but rather referred pain (Payne 1989b).

Pathophysiology

Tumor cells spread to bone mainly by the hematogenous route. In certain sites, direct invasion of bone may also occur. Oral or pharyngeal carcinomas may invade facial bones, and breast, lung, or esophageal tumors may directly involve the bony thorax. These tumors are usually ulcerating or pyogenic, since the bone periosteum is an effective barrier to closed noninfected cancers.

More than 80 percent of bone metastases are found in the axial skeleton because of the high distribution of red marrow in these bones. The spine, ribs, and pelvis are often the earliest site of metastases, whereas the skull, femora, humeri, scapulae, and sternum are involved later. Different primary tumors do not exhibit significant variation in their spread to bony sites, except that cancers of the prostate, bladder, cervix, and rectum tend to involve pelvic bones. Bone metastases are generally widespread by the time of their initial clinical presentation.

The destruction of bone is initially mediated by osteoclast-stimulating factors from the tumor or, more often, from the tumor-associated stroma or even the bone itself. In most carcinomas, the main factor is most likely a prostaglandin; in lymphoma and myeloma, it may be osteoclast-activating factor (OAF).

The relationship between bone invasion and bone pain is unclear. For example, 25 percent of patients with bone metastases have no symptoms; in the other 75 percent, however, pain is the main symptom. Postulated mechanisms that may cause pain from bone metastases include the following:

- stimulation of the nerve endings in the endosteum resulting from the destroyed bone's releasing a variety of chemical agents such as prostaglandin, bradykinin, substance P, or histamine;
- periosteal stretching by enlarging tumors;
- fractures; and
- extension of the tumor into the surrounding nerve and tissues.

Stimulation of endosteal nerve endings by released chemical agents is probably the dominant mechanism of bone pain from small metastases. As these metastases enlarge, stretching of the periosteum also contributes to the pain (Nielsen, Munro, and Tannock 1991).

Radiation Therapy

The management of a patient with painful bone metastases from advanced cancer generally involves more than one therapeutic approach to reach the goal of adequate pain control. When you have identified painful sites of bone metastases, consider localized radiotherapy. With this modality, palliation is achieved in 70 to 100 percent of patients (Poulsen et al. 1989). The available data suggest that, in most patients, local radiotherapy for painful localized bone metastases can be given as a single treatment of 8 Gy (Nielsen, Munro, and Tannock 1991; Poulsen et al. 1989).

The biologic basis by which radiotherapy relieves bone pain is unknown. This is underscored by the observation that some patients experience relief of pain within 48 hours of a single dose, whereas other patients do not achieve relief until two to eight weeks after treatment.

Radioactive isotopes, which deliver radiation systemically, have been administered for widespread involvement of bone. The bone-seeking isotope strontium-89 in several studies showed overall frequencies of pain relief of approximately 58 percent. However, the time to response is longer; therefore strontium-89 is not appropriate for the dying patient (Editorial, Strontium, 1990). Pain relief obtained with strontium-89 is probably similar to that achieved with hemibody radiation without the added risk of gastrointestinal or pulmonary toxicity.

Pharmacotherapy

Nonsteroidal Anti-inflammatory Drugs

Nonsteroidal anti-inflammatory drugs are often used for analgesic therapy for painful bone metastases. The NSAIDs, theoretically, block the synthesis of prostaglandin, which, in turn, obviates the role of prostaglandin in the destruction of bone and the stimulation of endosteal nerve endings. A study by Levick et al. (1988) compared the safety and efficacy of two dosages of naproxen sodium in 100 patients with bone pain due to metastatic cancer. In approximately 80 percent of the patients, either 550 mg of naproxen sodium orally three times a day or 275 mg orally three times a day provided relief from pain. Subsequent treatment on the high-dose regimen was more effective than the low-dose regimen in reducing the pain of bone metastases. Both regimens were equally tolerated; however, gastrointestinal complaints were reported in 7 percent on the low dose and 16 percent on the high dose.

In a related study, Toscani et al. (1989) used a subcutaneous continuous infusion of sodium naproxen in 14 patients with advanced cancer; these patients were unable to tolerate oral medication. Ten of the 14 patients (71 percent) had bone pain. The mean duration of the continuous subcutaneous infusion was 21 days, with a range of 7 to 112 days. In 4 patients, naproxen was combined with continuous morphine infusion, with a mean daily dose of naproxin of 1,100 mg. Ten patients were given naproxen infusion only at a mean daily dose of 1,375 mg. No pain or burning was noted at the infusion site, nor did intolerance or local or generalized reactions to naproxen occur. The same level of pain control achieved by prior oral naproxen administration was maintained for all patients.

Other NSAIDs, such as ketoprofen, indomethacin, and ibuprofen, may be effective in reducing pain due to metastatic bone disease (Payne 1989b).

BIPHOSPHONATES

Biphosphonates provide another method of treating bone metastases systemically. These agents, such as amidronate (APD), inhibit osteoclasts. In a randomized trial, Van Holten-Verzantvoort et al. (1987) studied the use of oral APD in 131 women with bone metastases from breast cancer. An interim analysis revealed a significant reduction in pathologic fractures and severe bone pain in the APD-treated group. Gastrointestinal side effects of APD, mainly nausea, led 8 percent of the patients to drop out of the study.

STEROIDS

Tannock et al. (1989) used low-dose prednisone (7.5 to 10 mg daily) to treat 37 male patients with prostatic cancer whose cancer had not been cured by prior therapy with estrogens and/or orchiectomy. The response to treatment was assessed by serial pain measurement instruments. Fourteen patients (38 percent) showed improvement in these scales used to measure pain at one month after starting prednisone, and 7 patients (19 percent) maintained this improvement for 3 to 30 months, with a median of 4 months. This reduction in pain was associated with an improvement in other dimensions of the quality of life as well as in overall well-being.

Summary

Bone metastases are common in patients with breast, lung, or prostate cancer and are often the source of severe, unrelenting pain. Local radiotherapy, given as a single treatment of 8 Gy, is effective palliation for painful localized bone metastases. The NSAIDs are the initial analgesic therapy to manage bone pain, but their usefulness is often limited by gastrointestinal toxicity. Low-dose prednisone may be useful in alleviating pain from metastatic bone disease in patients with prostatic cancer whose disease has failed to respond to hormonal manipulation. Further investigations are needed to clarify the role of the biphosphonates, such as APD, in palliative therapy for painful bone metastases.

Chapter 11

Surgery and Other Nonpharmacologic Interventions to Manage Pain

Surgery

Neurosurgical intervention provides an important alternative in the management of severe pain. The use of nerve blocks and neuroablative procedures to relieve pain has declined with the advent and refinement of the oral administration of opioids. Furthermore, neuroablation is not always permanent or always successful and has a high incidence of side effects (fig. 11.1). The indications for nerve blocks (Hanks and Justins 1992; Ferrer-Brechner 1989) (table 11.1) are

- pain responding to opioid analgesics, with an anticipated outcome of reducing doses and side effects and enhancing pain relief;
- pain not responding to opioid analgesics and control of psychologic factors;
- specific pains (e.g., those from pancreatic carcinoma and pathologic rib fractures); and
- the need for bodily functions important to the patient to be spared by the procedure.

Nondestructive nerve blocks involve the local injection of long-acting anesthetics, such as bupivacaine, or steroids and can be useful in determining the results of the destructive block intended. Local anesthetic can block central, epidural, peripheral (somatic and sympathetic), or visceral (celiac plexus) pain.

Destructive nerve blocks involve the injection of neurolytic solutions, such as alcohol and phenol, and the injection of freezing probes into nerves or ganglia. Neurolytic agents produce variable, nonselective nerve damage with a poor correlation between histologic damage and pain relief. The blocks are not permanent and last from hours to

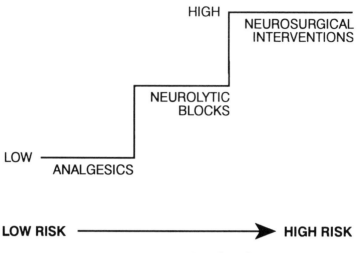

Figure 11.1   The Risk Related to Neuroablative Procedures

months (Ferrer-Brechner 1989). There is a high incidence of complications, including damage to adjacent structures, neuralgia, motor
weakness, and autonomic dysfunction (such as incontinence), which,
according to Hanks and Justins (1992), creates an unfavorable risk-
to-benefit ratio. In a divergent opinion from a different viewpoint
(namely, a pain clinic), Wells (1989) suggested that neurolytic procedures are underutilized. He reported that, in his experience as
Director of the Center for Pain Relief in Liverpool, United Kingdom,
83 percent of referred patients with cancer pain experienced pain
control with medication alone. Of the remaining 17 percent of patients, 13 percent were successfully treated by nerve block.

   More recently, Sharp and Stevens (1991) reported their experience
in using intraoperative celiac plexus block for pain relief in patients
with cancer of the pancreas. All patients had operative celiac plexus
block with absolute alcohol at the time of exploratory laparotomy for
biliary bypass, gastroenterostomy, or biopsy of tumor. Complete postoperative pain relief was obtained in 10 of the 12 patients, with 2
having partial pain relief. There were no operative complications related to the celiac plexus block. The mean postoperative survival was
3.5 months, and most patients had excellent pain relief for at least 2
months or until death.

   A short life expectancy does not limit the use of neurosurgical procedures (Hanks and Justins 1992; Wells 1989), but this approach is
associated with significant neurologic complications and morbidity.
Cordotomy is the most widely used and effective neuroablative proce-

Table 11.1   The Indications for Nerve
Blocks to Control Pain

Reduction in doses and side effects and en-
    hanced pain relief in opioid-responsive
    pain
Pain not responsive to opioid analgesics
Site-specific pain
    Pancreatic cancer
    Pathologic rib fractures
Preservation of important bodily functions

Sources: Ferrer-Brechner (1989); Hanks and
Justins (1992).

dure (Sundareson, DiGiacinto, and Hughes 1989); the pain fibers in
the anterolateral quadrant of the spinal cord are interrupted, thus
avoiding significant sensory and motor loss. Percutaneous cordotomy is
the most frequent procedure and consists of creating a lesion in the
anterolateral spinal cord at the C1-2 level by inserting a needle with
radiofrequency current (fig. 11.2).

Sundaresan, DiGiacinto, and Hughes (1989) summarized the results
of the five largest series of unilateral percutaneous cordotomies performed in cancer patients. In the 648 patients, the initial success rate
was high, ranging from 71 to 98 percent, but after one to two years
failures were common, with declining analgesia and, often, dysesthe-
sia. Morbidity ranged from 0 to 9 percent. Complications occurred, of
which respiratory depression was the most serious, since the respiratory fibers are located deep in the anterolateral quadrant. As noted by
Wells (1989), care must be taken in continuing oral opioids after percutaneous anterolateral cordotomy, since these drugs may enhance the
problem of postoperative respiratory depression. In addition to respiratory difficulties (range of 0 to 6 percent), long-term bladder dysfunction (range of 0 to 7 percent) and weakness (range of 0 to 10 percent)
were other complications of percutaneous cordotomies (Sundaresan,
DiGiacinto, and Hughes 1989).

Indications for percutaneous cordotomy (Hanks and Justins 1992;
Sundarson, DiGiacinto, and Hughes 1989; Wells 1989) are

- unilateral pain in patients when a reasonable attempt has been
  made to control the pain by the use of analgesic drugs,
- unilateral lower extremity pain due to lumbosacral plexopathy
  caused by rectal and gynecologic cancers, and
- mesothelioma.

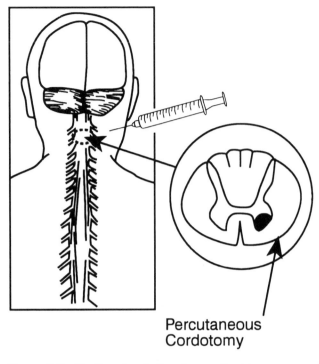

**Percutaneous
Cordotomy**

Figure 11.2   The Procedure for Percutaneous Cordotomy

Other, less frequently used surgical neuroablative procedures include the creation of a dorsal root entry zone lesion, midline commis-
sural myelotomy, dorsal rhizotomy, hypophysectomy, medullary trac-
totomy, and stereotactic procedures (Sundaresan, DiGiacinto, and
Hughes 1989).

Acupuncture

Acupuncture started in China during the Stone Ages. Flint needles
were used, and the evidence was recorded on tortoise shells. Huang Ti,
or the Yellow Emperor, reigned in approximately 2600 B.C. Ti wanted
to pass the secrets of medicine on to his sons and grandsons. To this
end, *The Yellow Emperor's Classic of Internal Medicine* (Veith 1972) was
written sometime between 475 and 221 B.C. The Yellow Emperor
thought that the balance of Yin and Yang, forces of opposite polarities

present in nature, was the basic principle of the entire universe. These forces—positive and negative, light and dark, masculine and feminine—should be present in appropriate amounts in each organ for healthy function.

Without question, the authors of the *Yellow Emperor's Classic* were strongly influenced by the beliefs of Lao-Tse, who had been born in 604 B.C. and from whom the religion of Taoism sprang. Taoism is based on scriptures from Lao-Tse called *Tao-te-Ching* or *The Book of Change*. Lao espoused the concept of Yin and Yang dynamism and balance in all aspects of life. Sickness is viewed as no more than an artificial separation from the life-giving and abundant energizers of the universe. To achieve health, the individual must restore the harmony and connection of these universal energizers with currents of the same energizers (Powell 1988).

The Chinese described a circulation of vital energy, Qi, with deep and superficial components. When Qi gels it causes life, but when dispersed it causes death. Qi travels throughout the body along meridians to nourish Yin and Yang of the various internal organs. These meridians are invisible lines joining a series of acupuncture points on the surface of the body.

By observation, the classification of acupuncture points has evolved over centuries. Any imbalance in the circulation of Qi could cause pain and disease. After taking a history and using a sophisticated pulse diagnosis, a physician could diagnose disease in 12 organs. The imbalance of energy could then be corrected by the insertion of needles into specifically chosen acupuncture points.

Despite centuries of use and decades of research, the precise mechanism of action of acupuncture in relieving pain remains unknown. As speculated by Filshie and Morrison (1988), acupuncture may work partly by involving natural pain inhibitory pathways such as endogenous opioids and by nonopioid neurohumeral mechanisms.

Few studies have been done on the use of acupuncture in the management of chronic pain in terminally ill patients. In the largest series, Filshie and Redman (1985) treated 183 cancer patients with acupuncture and found that more than half (52 percent) of the patients whose pain had not responded to conventional treatment were helped. The initial pain relief response to acupuncture was high (82 percent), but the relief was shortlived, from several hours to several days, in 30 percent of the responding patients. All patients required multiple treatments, often one to four times weekly. The investigators found acupuncture especially effective for pain due to vascular problems, dysesthetic conditions, muscle spasm, and metastatic bone disease.

Transcutaneous Electrical Nerve Stimulation

Transcutaneous electrical nerve stimulation (TENS) has been used for acute and chronic pain in a wide variety of settings, with varied results. TENS employs an electrical current applied to the skin to reduce or abolish the sensation of pain. Similar to acupuncture, TENS may stimulate the release of endogenous pain-relieving opioids. Unlike acupuncture, however, TENS may have longer-lasting effects.

In 1988, Librach and Rapson reviewed the medical literature over a 15-year period on the use of TENS in the treatment of cancer pain. They found scant research specifically investigating the use of TENS in cancer pain and found no investigative papers of this type in the literature on palliative care. One of the few descriptive studies (Avellamosa and West 1982) reported on 60 patients with cancer pain. After two weeks of treatment with TENS, there was an excellent response in 28 percent of patients, a fair response in 37 percent, and a failure to respond in 35 percent. After three months, however, these response rates were 15 percent, 18 percent, and 67 percent, respectively, showing a decline in response to placebo levels. The response of patients with bodily and extremity pain, especially upper limb pain, was better than the response of patients with pelvic or visceral pain. Overall, Librach and Rapson (1988) thought that the evidence documenting the effectiveness of TENS in cancer pain was spare and inconclusive.

Relaxation Techniques

The use of relaxation techniques in the acute pain setting is well appreciated (Acute Pain Management Guideline Panel 1992), but information is lacking on its use and efficacy in the dying patient with chronic pain. Some of the inherent difficulties in engaging these relaxation techniques in terminally ill patients are the cognitive function of the patient, length of time necessary to learn these approaches, and need for skilled personnel to teach them.

Summary

Nerve blocks and neuroablative procedures are important options in the management of pain. Nerve blocks are generally used for opioid-responsive pain when side effects are unmanageable and intolerable or for severe pain that does not respond to opioids. The use of an intraoperative celiac plexus block to relieve pain in patients with cancer of the pancreas is a good example of site-specific pain ablation. Radical neurosurgical procedures such as percutaneous cordotomy are rarely done, which attests to the effectiveness of oral opioids in controlling pain.

For other nonpharmacologic interventions—namely, acupuncture, transcutaneous electrical nerve stimulation, and relaxation techniques—scant scientific information exists to support their widespread use in the management of chronic pain in the dying patient.

PART III

The Management of Symptoms
during the Last Few Days

Chapter 12

The Final Moments

Death due to chronic illness, such as cancer, is rarely rapid. Dying usually lasts a few hours to days. It is a continuous process as the body and brain are unable to cope with hypoxia, malnutrition, electrolyte imbalance, tumor burden, and toxins that are not cleared from the body as hepatic and renal failure occur. Emotion, cognition, thinking, behavior, and autonomic function all slowly deteriorate and, in most cases, coma ensues before death.

Two roads to coma have been described in the dying patient: the high road and the low road. The low road is the most common and is a path of increasing sedation to coma and death. This path does not seem to be traumatic for patients, and survivors generally recall a peaceful death. If not controlled, the high road is much more traumatic, resembling the organic brain syndrome of delirium. Symptoms of this organic brain syndrome include restlessness, confusion, agitation, hallucinations, myoclonic jerks, seizures, and finally coma. A preterminal delirium can start as many as nine days before death. Over time, the symptoms often become increasing severe, and surviving family members frequently remember a terrible death even when the symptoms were well controlled up until the preterminal delirium (Ferris 1990).

Terminal Symptoms and Their Management

Lichter and Hunt (1990) designed a study to document the problems that arose during the last days in the life of terminally ill cancer patients and to record their frequency and the management used. Based on a pilot study, they chose a time frame of 48 hours because it was during this period that symptoms most commonly occurred in patients who had previously been comfortable.

Two hundred consecutive patients at the Te Omanga Hospice, in Lower Hutt, New Zealand, were studied. A patient record was established and maintained by the nurses when it was thought that the patient was likely to die or whenever terminal symptoms such as twitching, jerking, restlessness, agitation, and plucking were observed. The presence of other symptoms was also recorded, and observations were continued until the patient's death. In some cases, this was longer than 48 hours, and in these instances only the features occurring in the last 48 hours were analyzed.

The results of the study showed that 36 percent of patients experienced some problems in the last 48 hours of life. The great majority of patients (91.5 percent) died peacefully. Factors that interfered with a peaceful death in a few patients (8.5 percent) were hemorrhage and hemoptysis, respiratory distress, restlessness, pain, myocardial infarction, and regurgitation.

Slightly more than half (51 percent) of the patients experienced pain in the last 48 hours (table 12.1). Strict pain criteria were used, and every headache, backache, pressure area pain, movement pain, or transient discomfort noted at any time during the last 48 hours was recorded as pain. New pain was noted in 29.5 percent of the patients, and exacerbation of previously controlled pain occurred in 21.5 percent of patients.

Of all patients, 91 percent were on opioid analgesics and 25 percent were administered nonsteroidal anti-inflammatory drugs. Approximately the same number of patients required no change (39 percent) or an increased opioid dose (40 percent) during the last 48 hours. In only 12 percent was the dosage of opioids decreased. Pain was not completely controlled in 10 percent of patients, but no patient experienced persistent, severe pain.

Movement-related or disturbance pain was identified in 18 percent of the patients. This discomfort was noted even in comatose patients, who would moan or cry out when moved. It was suggested that this pain was related to joint stiffness and muscle weakness and that it can be eased by gentle passive movement at an earlier stage. Also, analgesics can be given before any major disturbance such as sponging.

Dyspnea occurred in 22 percent of the patients. The goal of treating terminal dyspnea is to relieve the perception of breathlessness. Dyspnea causing distress is generally associated with tachypnea accompanied by anxiety. A draft of cool air is helpful in alleviating this shortness of breath and can be achieved by opening a window or using a fan. It is thought that the perception of breathlessness is altered by stimulating receptors in the distribution of the trigeminal nerve in the cheek. Also, the passage of cool air into the nasal cavity relieves dyspnea by further stimulating other trigeminal nerve receptors in the nasopharynx. If additional measures are needed, a benzodiazepine can

Table 12.1 The Frequency of Symptoms and Their Management during the Last 48 Hours of Life

Symptom (Frequency)	Management
Noisy and moist breathing (56%)	Atropine or scopolamine (0.4 mg repeated every 4–8h as needed) along with morphine (10–15 mg)
	Suctioning, change of position, and reassurance
Pain (51%)	Adjustment in opioid dosage
Restlessness and agitation (42%)	Methotrimeprazine (25–50 mg IM[a] every 4h as required)
	Diazepam (5–10 mg)
	Chlorpromazine (50 mg every 4 to 8h)
	Midazolam (10 mg stat dose and then starting dose of 30 mg/day using continuous infusion)
	Lorazepam (sublingually in doses of 1–2 mg every hour as needed)
Urinary incontinence (32%) and retention (21%)	Padding
	Male external catheter
	Indwelling catheter
Difficulty swallowing (29%)	Rectal administration of drugs
	Continuous infusion of medications, preferably subcutaneous, via pump device
Dyspnea (22%)	Reassurance
	Bedside fan
	Diazepam (5–10 mg stat dose and then 5–20 mg at night)
	Morphine (5–10 mg every 4h or doses of morphine titrated to achieve a respiratory rate of 15–20 respirations/min)
Nausea and vomiting (14%)	Antiemetics, such as haloperidol, administered by continuous infusion
Sweating and feeling of heat (14%)	Steroids
	Indomethacin (100 mg rectally)
Muscle twitching, jerking, and plucking (12%)	Diazepam
	Midazolam (5 mg stat dose and starting dose of 10 mg/day by continuous infusion as muscle relaxant; 5 mg stat dose and starting dose of 20 mg/day by continuous infusion for multifocal myoclonus)
Confusion (9%)	Reassurance
	Haloperidol (5–10 mg IM stat dose, then oral or IM 5–15 mg daily)
	Chlorpromazine (50 mg)

Sources: Lichter and Hunt (1990); Saunders (1982); McNamara, Minton, and Twycross (1991).
[a] IM, intramuscular.

be administered. The perception of breathlessness can also be relieved by reducing the rate of breathing to a comfortable level using morphine. The dose of morphine is titrated against the respiratory rate to obtain a rate of 15 to 20 respirations per minute. Patients already receiving morphine for pain usually require an approximately 50 percent increase in dose to achieve a suitable reduction in respiratory rate. Of the 22 percent of patients experiencing terminal dyspnea, all but 2 percent responded to treatment with morphine and a benzodiazepine, usually very promptly.

Noisy and moist breathing was present in 56 percent of the patients. Although not distressful to the patient, moist respirations or the death rattle was troubling to relatives and caregivers. Anticholinergic drugs such as atropine or scopolamine (0.4 mg) were effective if existing secretions in the back of the throat were first cleared. Noisy respiration requiring medication was noted in 25 percent of patients. Anticholinergic drugs were immediately successful in 94 percent of these patients, and 6 percent required repeated doses. A further 31 percent needed only nursing interventions, which included suctioning, change of position, and reassurance.

Nausea and vomiting was noted in only 14 percent of the patients. In 6 percent it was a continuation or exacerbation of previously existing nausea and vomiting, and in 8 percent it was a new symptom. For exacerbations, increases in continuously infused antiemetics were needed. In some patients, treatment of constipation relieved this symptom.

Nine percent of the patients experienced confusion in the last 48 hours. Confusion was best managed by reassurance. Restraints were not used; instead, constant supervision was maintained. When the confusion was marked, drug treatment was added. Haloperidol (5 to 10 mg intramuscular immediately and then oral administration, or intramuscular 5 to 15 mg daily) was helpful, especially in the presence of hallucinations or paranoia. Benzodiazepines were useful when the patient was restless and agitated, although they may have a paradoxical effect and increase restlessness. Chlorpromazine (dose of 50 to 100 mg) was sometimes successful when haloperidol failed and was particularly useful when sedation was needed.

Restlessness and agitation occurred frequently (42 percent). For relieving restlessness, methotrimeprazine (25 to 50 mg given intramuscularly and repeated every four hours as needed), which has both analgesic and antiemetic properties, was used. If the restlessness was not controlled, the addition of a benzodiazepine such as diazepam was often effective. An alternate was chlorpromazine. These drugs singly or in combination relieved restlessness in all patients. In 5 percent of patients, a change of medication was successful when the drug of first choice was not effective.

Muscle twitching and jerking was identified in 12 percent of the patients. The treatment of choice was benzodiazepines and anticonvulsants, and good relief was obtained in all patients.

Urinary incontinence and the retention of urine were recorded in 32 percent and 21 percent of the patients, respectively. An indwelling catheter was used in 44 percent, and a male external catheter was used in 4 percent. A common cause of difficulty of micturition was the presence of rectal feces, which was managed by suppository, enema, or manual removal.

Sweating occurred in 14 percent of the patients and was usually managed with steroids and indomethacin.

Finally, the authors studied the time duration of consciousness. Thirty percent of the patients were conscious until death, 38 percent became unconscious 0 to 12 hours before death, 24 percent became unconscious 12 to 24 hours before death, 7 percent became unconscious 24 to 48 hours before death, and 1 percent were unconscious for more than 48 hours.

SUBLINGUAL LORAZEPAM

To prevent hospitalization and maintain the patient at home, sublingual lorazepam and continuous subcutaneous infusions of midazolam have been used to control restlessness and other terminal symptoms. Ferris (1990) suggested the use of sublingual lorazepam as an alternative to haloperidol in dying patients unable to swallow. This route also obviates the need for intermittent painful injections and is well suited for the home care setting. Lorazepam is given sublingually in dosages of 1 to 2 mg every hour as needed with a few drops of water, and the dosage is increased to 2 to 4 mg every hour as needed. Sedation occurs in most patients after a few milligrams, and subsequent doses can be administered when symptoms recur.

MIDAZOLAM

Amesbury and Dunphy (1989) used continuous subcutaneous infusions of midazolam to manage terminal restlessness in six patients cared for at home. Midazolam is a short-acting, water-soluble benzodiazepine used as the sole induction agent, in some cases, for anesthesia and frequently used for sedation, especially where amnesia is desirable. All six patients had advanced cancer. The mean patient age was 65 years, with a range of 45 to 84 years. A continuous infusion pump was used because the patients were experiencing episodes of reduced consciousness that made it difficult to swallow medication for pain and/or nausea and vomiting. In all cases, the infusion was continued until death, with a mean duration of 64 hours and a range of 24 to 216 hours. The mean total daily dose of midazolam was 30 mg, with a range of 20 to 40 mg. When the midazolam infusion was added, the restlessness ceased in all cases. No side effects were noted with its use in this setting.

In a related paper, McNamara, Minton, and Twycross (1991) retrospectively studied the use of midazolam in 104 terminal patients. In 3 patients midazolam was administered intravenously as sedation for minor procedures; in 1 patient it was used intermittently subcutaneously as short-term sedation pending epidural analgesia. The 100 remaining patients received midazolam by continuous subcutaneous infusion for terminal agitation (61), muscle stiffness (27), multifocal myoclonus (7), and seizure prophylaxis (5). The median age of these 100 patients was 69 years, with a range of 26 to 89 years. The median dose was 30 mg/24 hours, and only 6 of 61 patients with terminal agitation required more than 100 mg/24 hours. No clinically relevant episodes of respiratory depression occurred, despite the fact that midazolam was often given in conjunction with opioids. No skin irritation was noted, even at the highest dose used, 240 mg/24 hours.

In the investigator's experience, midazolam was a safe and effective drug in the terminal setting. Based on this, they offered the following guidelines for the use of midazolam:

- as a muscle relaxant (5 mg stat dose, starting infusion rate of 10 mg/24 hours, common range of 10 to 30 mg/24 hours);
- for terminal agitation (10 mg stat dose, starting infusion rate of 30 mg/24 hours, common range of 30 to 60 mg/24 hours);
- as an anticonvulsant, including multifocal myoclonus (5 mg stat dose, starting infusion rate of 20 mg/24 hours, common range of 20 to 40 mg).

Drug-induced Terminal Sedation

As part of the National Hospice Study (NHS), Morris et al. (1986) studied the quality of life of terminally ill cancer patients. They collected data from two samples of cancer patients for the last 13 weeks of their lives. One sample consisted of patients followed in two hospital-based palliative care units in Montreal, Canada, as part of a controlled study by the McGill Cancer Center. The other sample comprised patients in six hospices in the United States participating in the National Hospice Study project funded by the Health Care Financing Administration.

Using this information, the investigators tested a series of hypotheses concerning the quality of life during the final 13 weeks. They proposed two general clinical scenarios. In the first, they postulated that the patient experienced a significant loss of quality of life over some weeks, which resulted in the unrelenting picture of functional decline and symptomatic distress. In the second, a loss of quality of life was depicted as sudden and lasting the final one to two weeks. A wide array of measures of the quality of life were used in the study.

Not surprisingly, the data supported the second scenario: declines in the quality of life varied as a function of the patient's proximity to death, with rapid decline being limited to the last one to three weeks of life. Many patients were in extreme pain some nine weeks before death, whereas many others had little or no pain. As death approached, the distribution of patients in pain changed little, and there was no rapid rise in either the average levels of pain or the number of patients with extreme pain during the last one to three weeks of life. Finally, some 20 percent of the patients did not fall into the categories of having a very low quality of life, even in the week before death.

The finding of no dramatic change in pain as death approached, reported by Morris et al. (1986), was also reported by Higginson and McCarthy (1989). These latter investigators studied the symptoms of 86 patients referred to a district terminal care support team. Pain was the most common severe symptom, occurring in a little less than half of the referred patients. Pain control was improved after one week of care by the support team, and further improvement was maintained until death, with no patient dying in severe pain.

One possible conclusion from these studies is that the vast majority of terminally ill cancer patients are dying pain-free after a short downhill clinical course that lasts only a few weeks. However, if this is valid, why the recent appearance in the medical literature of three articles (Fainsinger et al. 1991; Greene and Davis 1991; Ventafridda, Ripamonti, DeConno, et al. 1990) on the topic of terminal sedation for uncontrolled symptoms? One answer may be that the results of scientific inquiry do not always reflect the realities of terminal care. Another answer may be confusion regarding terminology such as *pain* and *suffering*, the definition of symptoms, and the like.

Ventafridda, Ripamonti, DeConno, et al. (1990) studied 120 terminal cancer patients prospectively entering a home care program organized by the Palliative Care Division of the National Cancer Institute of Milan. The home care team consisted of five physicians, seven registered nurses, one psychologist, one social worker, and approximately one hundred volunteers. All patients were treated for pain based on the World Health Organization guidelines. The intensity of symptoms was assessed by an endurable/unendurable scale as reported by the patient. When symptoms could not be relieved through specific or symptomatic treatment, the dosages of opioids (morphine, methadone) and/or strong tranquilizers (diazepam, chlorpromazine, haloperidol) were gradually increased until the symptoms were controlled. Before entry into the study, the patients and families were informed that it is always possible to control symptoms but that sometimes this can be accomplished only by reducing the patients' level of consciousness. Both patients and families expressed their consent to this therapeutic approach.

Of the 120 patients, 73 were men and 47 were women, with a median age of 65.5 years. Lung cancer was the most common diagnosis. During the entire period of home care, there were 123 episodes of symptoms characterized by the patients as unendurable. In slightly more than one-third of the patients, the symptoms were controlled through therapeutic intervention by the home care physician. These controllable symptoms included pain (60 percent) and dyspnea (40 percent). However, symptoms were not controlled in 52 percent of the patients despite active symptomatic treatment. These symptoms appeared on average two days before death. Symptom control in these patients was possible only by increasing the dosages of drugs, predominantly opioids and tranquilizers, until sedation or sleep occurred. This lowered level of consciousness was maintained until death and was carried out with the advance permission of the patient or on an ad hoc basis.

Of the 63 patients who required sedation for uncontrollable symptoms, 75 percent had only one symptom, 24 percent had two, and 1 percent had three. The majority of patients had either dyspnea (41 percent) or pain (39 percent), with fewer patients experiencing delirium (14 percent) or vomiting (6 percent). Dyspnea was most frequent in patients with lung and head and neck cancers, whereas pain occurred in patients with breast, gastrointestinal tract, colorectal, and male genitourinary tract cancers. Vomiting was seen in patients with cancer of the female genitourinary tract.

The causes of these uncontrolled symptoms were also investigated. In slightly more than half of the cases with dyspnea, massive tumor invasion of the lung parenchyma was found. Pain was related to bone involvement in one-third of the cases, and delirium was frequently related to the presence of brain metastases. Finally, vomiting generally was correlated with the occurrence of inoperable gastrointestinal tract obstruction.

From the start of home care, the median length of survival was 25 days for patients in whom sedation was necessary and 23 days for the other patients. This difference was not statistically significant.

The investigators involved in this study thought that their results highlighted important information that has been neglected in the published literature, that is, more than 50 percent of patients with terminal cancer will die with physical suffering that can be controlled only by sedation. Furthermore, the authors speculated that the onset of unendurable and uncontrollable symptoms was a good prognosticator of imminent death. Finally, the authors did address, to some degree, the ethical question of this approach and thought that it was correct only if the patient's wishes were respected.

In a related article, Greene and Davis (1991) reported their experience with 17 terminally ill patients in whom they used continuous intravenous barbiturates to control symptoms. The authors did a retrospective review of patients with terminal cancer in their community-based urology practice. During the years 1975 to 1989, 17 patients with terminal cancer who were very close to death were identified. All attempts at curative treatment had been exhausted, and standard methods of palliative therapy were insufficient. The 17 patients ranged in age from 56 to 86 years, with a mean of 69. The tumor sites included prostate (8), bladder (5), kidney (2), colon (1), and pancreas (1). Symptoms included pain in bone and soft tissue, prolonged vomiting, abdominal distension, seizures, fecal emesis, retention of urine, and restlessness. Fifteen of these 17 patients were experiencing some degree of pain.

Prerequisites for intravenous barbiturate therapy included the following.

- The patient had terminal cancer.
- All other palliative treatments were exhausted.
- Death was imminent, that is, likely to occur within hours or days.
- A do-not-resuscitate order was in effect.
- The patient and all family members were in agreement.
- A family member was in attendance at the bedside at all times.

In the first nine patients, amobarbital sodium, a short- to intermediate-acting barbiturate, was used. Initial dosages ranged from 20 to 215 mg/hour, depending on the patient's weight and overall condition. An average dosage of 218 mg/hour was employed. Thiopental sodium, an ultrashort-acting barbiturate, was administered to the last eight patients and was preferred because of its short half-life and the ease with which the dosage could be controlled. The mean dosage of thiopental required was 107 mg/hour. Unfortunately, the investigators did not use any objective parameters to measure the patient's level of consciousness other than simple clinical observation. Four patients died without total somnolence, but somnolence developed over 6 to 24 hours in the remaining 13 patients. This reduced level of consciousness lasted 2 hours to four days, averaging 23 hours. According to the investigators, the patients all died peacefully in their sleep.

The use of a single-agent barbiturate allowed the investigators to induce somnolence or pharmacologic hypnosis to dissociate the patient's consciousness from severe symptoms. To the investigators, it seemed logical to achieve a somnolent effect with the use of a hypnotic agent rather than to increase an opioid toward its limit of toxicity to produce sedation. Continuous intravenous barbiturate is accepted therapy in other areas of medical practice, such as in the control of intubated patients receiving ventilatory support. As in Ventafridda, Ripamonti, DeConno, et al.'s (1990) study, sedation therapy was done with the consent of the patients and families.

Addressing the issue of the appropriateness of physician-assisted suicide for terminally ill patients, Greene and Davis (1991) observed that, when symptom control is successful, cancer patients find no need to ask for euthanasia as a means of escape. Furthermore, the investigators thought that any shortening of life was incident to their objective of relieving suffering in situations where the extension of life had no meaning.

More recently and in response to the study by Ventafridda, Ripamonti, DeConno, et al. (1990), Fainsinger et al. (1991) reported their experience with terminal sedation to control symptoms at the Edmonton General Hospital. These investigators retrospectively reviewed 100 consecutive patients admitted for six days or more to a 14-bed palliative care unit. Of the 100 patients, 51 were men and 49 were women, with a mean age of 62 years. Carcinoma of the gastrointestinal tract was the most common diagnosis, and the mean duration of admission was 40 days. A review of patient charts was done to collect information on major symptoms requiring treatment, symptom control at admission and during each of the last seven days of life, drugs used, and changes that may have contributed to sedation. Of the 100 patients, 99 needed treatment for pain, 71 for nausea, 46 for dyspnea, and 39 for delirium. Visual analog scores were done twice daily on all patients to assess pain and symptoms. The evaluation of patient records and changes in medication (with particular reference to sedating drugs, increasing doses, and changes in level of consciousness) revealed that 6 of 99 patients (6 percent) with pain and 10 of 39 patients (26 percent) with delirium required increased treatment, likely resulting in their sedation to an unresponsive state during the last days of life. Thus, the authors concluded, only 16 of 100 patients (16 percent) required treatment for pain and delirium that would have caused sedation to achieve control of symptoms.

Although the characteristics of the patients in these two studies (Fainsinger et al. 1991; Ventafridda, Ripamonti, DeConno, et al. 1990) are similar, the results are strikingly different; that is, 52 percent versus 16 percent of terminally ill patients required sedation for symptom control. Also, the studies used differing methods. Ventafridda, Ripamonti, DeConno, et al. (1990) prospectively studied their patients, whereas Fainsinger et al. (1991) opted for a retrospective review of the patients' charts. The inherent weakness of this retrospective approach may well explain the disparity in the findings of these two investigations.

As noted by Roy (1991) in an editorial commenting on Ventafridda, Ripamonti, DeConno, et al.'s study, this question of sedation-induced unconsciousness raises many issues, including ethical ones. Roy (1991) argued that the agitated and restless patient does little to prepare himself or herself and the family for death. In this instance, death in a sleep and forgetting state can bring comfort and peace. On the other hand, the use of drugs as a blunderbuss at the end of life would be to write off patients at the very moment they need the most sensitive and competent care.

Summary

In the dying patient, death is preceded by either progressive sedation or the development of the organic brain syndrome, delirium. More than one-third of dying patients experience some difficulties during their last 48 hours of life, with noisy and moist breathing, pain, and agitation and restlessness being the most common. The great majority of these symptoms can be managed by reassurance or drug intervention. Sublingual lorazepam and the continuous subcutaneous infusion of midazolam are effective in controlling terminal restlessness.

A disparity exists in the medical literature regarding the extent of control of a patient's symptoms just before death. According to Ventafridda, Ripamonti, DeConno, et al. (1990), more than half of the patients they studied required drug-induced sedation to control symptoms, whereas Fainsinger et al. (1991) found that only 16 percent of their patients needed terminal sedation. In a related study, Greene and

Davis (1991) reported the use of barbiturate-induced sedation in 17 patients over a 15-year period to alleviate uncontrolled physical suffering shortly before death. Clearly, more research and open discussion of this topic are needed to define more fully the appropriateness of this approach and to delineate how close terminal sedation comes to the line of euthanasia.

Chapter 13

Issues Concerning the Sustaining of Life

Do Not Resuscitate

In the past several years, intense interest has focused on the complexities of the decision not to resuscitate. The prerogative not to resuscitate is the patient's, and this instruction means that, if cardiac and/or pulmonary arrest occurs, no therapeutic attempt is made to reverse these events, and death ensues. In 1983, the President's Commission for the study of Ethical Problems in Medicine and Biomedical and Behavioral Research raised three critical points: (1) resuscitation is a very painful and intrusive procedure; (2) efforts to resuscitate a dying patient are successful in only approximately one attempt in three and, of those patients who survive initial resuscitation efforts, only one-third are eventually discharged (those who are able to return home are often significantly impaired); and (3) the success of resuscitation efforts is generally difficult to assess without carrying out the full range of procedures. These facts suggest that physicians who carry out less aggressive efforts because they did not thoroughly consider the resuscitation decision ahead of time may not be acting in their patients' best interests.

Based on their deliberations, the President's Commission made three chief recommendations for the development of policies on resuscitation. (1) Hospitals should develop explicit policies on the practice of writing and implementing do-not-resuscitate (DNR) orders. (2) Hospital policies should recognize the need for balanced protection of the patients and respect the right of a competent patient to make an informed choice. (3) Hospital policies should provide a means for appropriate resolution of conflicts and also mandate internal review. In addition to these broad guidelines, the report noted that much of medical practice is now governed by private and independent organizations, such as the Joint Commission on Accreditation of Healthcare Organizations (JCAHO), that bear a responsibility to encourage sound decisions regarding resuscitation. The President's Commission specifically suggested that, to be accredited, hospitals should at least be required to have a general policy regarding resuscitation, preferably one that addresses the three points cited above.

In response to these recommendations as well as those from other health care organizations such as the American Hospital Association and the American Medical Association, the JCAHO did a DNR policy survey in 1986. The purposes of this study were to determine the extent of use, nature, and implementation of DNR policies. Additional data identified common problems encountered in implementing DNR policies in addition to methods of resolving conflicts in the use of DNR orders. Enck et al. (1988) reported the clinically relevant results of this 1986 study, with a special comparative analysis of the hospice data.

A cross-sectional, random sample of health care organizations stratified by setting (acute care hospitals, psychiatric hospitals, long-term care facilities, hospices) was identified. A mail survey questionnaire was then sent to these 2,021 health care organizations; a response rate of 61 percent was reached, with a confidence interval of 95 percent. The hospice sample size was 504, with a 62 percent response rate (312 hospices).

Overall, the results revealed variability across all settings in the extent of having formal, informal, and no DNR policies: 31 percent had a formal policy, 28 percent had an informal policy, and 41 percent had no policy. Hospices ranked second to acute care hospitals in having formal DNR policies (43 percent and 57 percent, respectively) (table 13.1).

In those hospices with a formal policy, DNR orders were written most often (90 percent) on patients with cancer, followed, in decreasing frequency, by patients with renal failure, stroke, congestive heart fail-

Table 13.1   Do-Not-Resuscitate Treatment Policy by Health Care Setting

	% of Institutions		
Health Care Setting	Formal	Informal	None
Acute care	57	29	14
Hospice care	43	20	38
Long-term care	20	30	50
Psychiatric care	11	8	80
Total (all settings)	31	28	41

Source: Enck et al. (1988).

ure, Alzheimer disease and related disorders, coronary artery disease, acute myocardial infarction, and pneumonia.

If a decision was made for no cardiopulmonary resuscitation (CPR), defibrillation, intubation/ventilation, and medication were allowed in 69 percent of hospices and 79 percent of other settings with a formal DNR policy. Thus, in more than half the hospices with a formal DNR policy, resuscitation measures other than CPR were included in the policy.

Approximately one-fourth of hospices with a formal DNR policy addressed the withholding and/or withdrawal of treatments and interventions other than CPR. Hospices lacking a formal DNR policy, however, addressed these areas much less often (14 percent). Generally, in both groups these policies were in the following clinical areas: use of ventilator, nutrition/hydration, antibiotic therapy, and care of compromised infants.

In hospices with either formal, written DNR policies or informal, implicit policies, the need for continuing education on this topic for nursing and medical staffs was the commonest implementation problem. It was striking that one-third of the respondants reported nursing and medical staff conflict as a problem of implementation (table 13.2).

If conflicts in the use of DNR orders arose, resolution most often occurred by an informal meeting with family/guardian (68 percent). The use of the judicial system was the lowest rated mechanism for resolving conflict (8 percent). Also, the conflict resolution process gen-

Table 13.2 The Frequency of Common Problems Encountered in Implementing Do-Not-Resuscitate (DNR) Policies

Problem	Frequency (%)
Need for continuing education on this topic for nursing and medical staffs	41
Definition of relationships of DNR to other treatments	38
Conflict between nursing and medical staffs as to appropriateness of DNR orders	33
Obtaining of medical staff agreement/compliance with DNR policies	27
Legal issues	26
Obtaining of attending physician countersignature in required time frame	24
Inability to establish functioning ethics/DNR-related committee	18
Difficulty getting nursing staff to accept policies	10

Source: Enck et al. (1988).

erally used a consultant for a second opinion regarding a patient's treatment or prognosis. In more than 90 percent of the responses, physicians in an appropriate specialty were identified as the consultants, followed by a nursing representative, clergy/spiritual counselor, medical director of a special unit, psychosocial worker, attorney, chief of staff, patient advocate, and ethicist/philosopher.

The ideal of providing maximal comfort to the dying patient through all phases of the terminal illness is a cornerstone of hospice care. Therefore, the investigators were surprised to find that only 43 percent of the hospices surveyed had a formal written policy on DNR. Furthermore, only one in five hospices had an informal policy, and more than one-third had no policy on DNR at all. On the other hand, hospices with a formal policy more clearly reflected the relationship of DNR to the patient's overall management than did acute, psychiatric, and long-term care settings. This critical insight into the complex role of DNR in patient care further strengthens the need for hospices to go through the process of developing these DNR policies, noted the authors.

As defined by Evans and Brody (1985), efforts at resuscitation may be divided into three categories: all available life-sustaining measures, all such measures except intubation, and basic CPR without active medications and intubation. In their study of three teaching hospitals, they reported that less than full resuscitation efforts were made in 43 percent of cases where a final decision to resuscitate had not been made.

In an effort to delineate further the resuscitation efforts in hospice care, Enck et al. (1988) inquired about the use of other resuscitation measures, namely, defibrillation, intubation/ventilation, and chemical treatment in patients where basic cardiopulmonary resuscitation was not performed. More than half allowed the use of these therapeutic interventions as part of a formal DNR policy, thus extending the observation of Evans and Body (1985) that the DNR decision in the clinical setting is more often broad than it is narrow in scope.

Hospices with a formal DNR policy addressed the areas of withholding and/or withdrawing treatments more often than did hospices without such formal policies. The use of a ventilator and nutrition/hydration were commonly cited clinical areas. Thus, those programs that went through the DNR decision-making process were also able to extend this into other areas, such as withholding or stopping interventions other than CPR (Enck et al. 1988).

In addressing the issue of survival of cancer patients after CPR, Faber-Langendoen (1991) reviewed all studies published from 1980 to 1989 that reported survival after CPR. Nine of these studies specifically included data on patients with cancer, and not all studies separated patients with metastatic cancer from those with localized disease. Fewer patients (3 percent) with cancer survived to hospital discharge than did patients with other diseases (12 percent). Of these survivors, all had localized disease. There were no survivors in any study among patients with metastatic cancer. In discussing these findings, Faber-Langendoen (1991) noted that, although communication and patient autonomy are critically important, physicians must not propose treatments that do not work, and CPR does not work in patients with metastatic cancer.

Indeed, not only patient communication and autonomy but also having the correct diagnosis of terminal cancer is of utmost importance. To this end, Rees, Dover, and Low-Beer (1987) reported the misdiagnosis of terminal cancer in four patients referred for supportive care. For a variety of reasons, each of these patients was wrongly labeled as having cancer when, in fact, nonmalignant diseases accounted for their failing health. When appropriately treated, they lived 18 months to 6+ years.

To identify the wishes of patients for information, participation in decision making, and life-sustaining treatment as well as to determine whether these wishes are stable over time, Silverstein et al. (1991) conducted a prospective survey of 38 patients with an established diagnosis of ALS at the University of Chicago Motor Neuron Disease Clinic. A baseline survey was done, and then the survey was repeated at six-month intervals. The interview format was used with a structured questionnaire. Twenty-five men and 13 women with an average age of 54 years participated in the study. The investigators found that preferences for CPR in two hypothetical circumstances, involving pneumonia, mechanical ventilation, and cardiac arrest, were much less stable over time than were desires for information and participation in decision making. Some patients changed their wishes from not wanting CPR to wanting it, whereas other patients changed their minds and no longer wanted to be resuscitated. Changes were not related to the patients' clinical or demographic characteristics. The authors concluded that, because many patients with ALS change their desires for life-sustaining treatment, advance directives for end-of-life care must be reevaluated periodically.

Organizations such as the American Medical Association have provided guidelines for the appropriate use of DNR orders (Council on Ethical and Judicial Affairs 1991), which urge that these decisions be made openly. In an accompanying editorial, Lo (1991) offered some suggestions that may be helpful for physicians and patients in discussions about DNR orders. First, physicians should raise the subject of

DNR in a straightforward manner and explain what CPR involves. Second, physicians must provide enough information for patients to make informed decisions. This discussion can be explicit without being blunt or threatening. Third, physicians should offer specific recommendations but also give the patient appropriate choices. Fourth, physicians should place CPR discussions in a positive context of supportive care while allaying patients' fear of pain and abandonment. Fifth, discussions about CPR need to be repeated, allowing the patients and families enough time to think about the issues and to deal with their emotions. Sixth, physicians can improve their skill in discussing DNR orders.

Advance Directives

In the wake of the Cruzan case, which renewed national interest in using advance directives to avoid unwanted medical interventions, President Bush signed the Patient Self-Determination Act (PSDA) on November 5, 1990, and it went into effect on December 1, 1991. As a requirement for Medicare and Medicaid payment, the PSDA dictates that hospitals, skilled nursing facilities, home health agencies, hospices, and health maintenance organizations

- develop written policies regarding advance directives;
- ask all new patients whether they have prepared an advance directive, such as a living will or durable power of attorney, and include this information on the patient's chart;
- give patients written materials regarding the institution's policies on advance directives and the patient's rights (under applicable state law) to prepare such documents; and
- educate the community and the institutional staff regarding advance directives (Greco et al. 1991).

Although the PSDA is new and experience with its implementation and use is limited, reservations about it are already being expressed. Wolf et al. (1991) voiced concern that advance directives may wrongly be viewed as the only way to make future treatment decisions and may, furthermore, reduce the discussion of therapeutic alternatives and directives to a bureaucratic process dominated by forms and brochures. The authors stressed the importance of periodic review of advance directives and thought that the PSDA's requirement should be seen as a catalyst for broader innovation to integrate advance directives into good patient care.

Enacting the PSDA, however, does not ensure that all adults will prepare or periodically update advance directives before a catastrophic illness. In this instance, there is often strong societal pressure in favor of preserving life regardless of the prognosis for recovery. Therefore, in many cases, the absence of an advance directive results in an implicit decision to start or continue life-sustaining treatment. This societal standard, however, conflicts with a growing body of evidence that most people do not want life-sustaining treatment if they become permanently unconscious or terminally ill. One possible solution for this dilemma would be for health care facilities to develop formal treatment guidelines based on the consensus of the lay and the medical communities (Greco et al. 1991).

The withdrawal of nutrition and hydration remains a controversial issue. Some are critical of stopping this form of treatment, which is considered a basic link between one person and another. The withdrawal of nutrition and hydration may also be perceived as directly hastening the death of a patient (Duffy 1992). In this circumstance, advance directives may not be helpful because of quirks of state law. Under Illinois law, for example, living wills do not apply to the withdrawal of nutrition and hydration (Blum 1990).

Summary

Hospices and other health care organizations caring for dying patients need to develop formal DNR policies, since this decision-making process is easily extended into other areas, such as withholding or stopping interventions other than CPR. The importance of addressing the DNR issue is highlighted by a study (Faber-Langendoen 1991) that found no survivors after CPR in patients with metastatic cancer. On the other hand, before a DNR decision is made regarding a terminally ill cancer patient, the diagnosis must be correct (Rees, Dover, and Low-Beer 1987). Critical to making a DNR order is a frank and open discussion between the patient and the physician. This discussion should be repeated periodically, since some patients change their minds, as noted in patients with ALS (Silverstein et al. 1991).

Advance directives are a new requirement for Medicare and Medicaid reimbursement. Therefore, little experience has been reported from which to draw firm conclusions.

References

Acute Pain Management Guideline Panel. 1992. Options to prevent and control postoperative pain. In *Acute pain management: Operative or medical procedures and trauma. Clinical Practice Guideline*, 15–26. Rockville, Md.: Agency for Health Care Policy and Research, Public Health Service, U.S. Department of Health and Human Services.

Ahlquist, D. A., C. J. Gostout, T. R. Viggiano, R. K. Balm, P. C. Pairolero, V. S. Hench, and A. R. Zinsmeister. 1987. Endoscopic laser palliation of malignant dysphagia: A prospective study. *Mayo Clinic Proceedings* 62:867–74.

Allan, S. G. 1988. Emesis in the patient with advanced cancer. *Palliative Medicine* 2:89–100.

Allman, R. M. 1989. Pressure ulcers among the elderly. *New England Journal of Medicine* 320:850–53.

Allman, R. M., C. L. Laprade, L. B. Noel, J. M. Walker, C. A. Moorer, M. R. Dear, and C. R. Smith. 1986. Pressure sores among hospitalized patients. *Annals of Internal Medicine* 105:337–42.

Allman, R. M., J. M. Walker, M. K. Hart, C. A. Laprade, L. B. Noel, and C. R. Smith. 1987. Air-fluidized beds or conventional therapy for pressure sores. *Annals of Internal Medicine* 107:641–48.

American College of Physicians. 1989. Parenteral nutrition in patients receiving cancer chemotherapy. *Annals of Internal Medicine* 110:734–36.

Amesbury, B. D. W., and K. P. Dunphy. 1989. The use of subcutaneous midazolam in the home care setting. *Palliative Medicine* 3:299–301.

Andrews, M. R., and A. M. Levine. 1989. Dehydration in the terminal patient: Perception of hospice nurses. *American Journal of Hospice Care* 6:31–34.

Angell, M. 1982. The quality of mercy. *New England Journal of Medicine* 306:98–99.

Aranha, G. V., F. A. Folk, and H. B. Greenlee. 1981. Surgical palliation of small bowel obstruction due to metastatic cancer. *American Surgeon* 47:99–102.

Ashby, M., and B. Stoffell. 1991. Therapeutic ratio and defined phases: Proposal of ethical framework for palliative care. *British Medical Journal* 302:1322–24.

Ashford, R., G. Plant, J. Maher, and L. Teare. 1984. Double-blind trial of metronidazole in malodorous ulcerating tumors. *Lancet* 1:1232–33.

Avellamosa, A. M., and C. R. West. 1982. Experience with transcutaneous nerve stimulation for relief of intractable pain in cancer patients. *Journal of Medicine* 13:203–13.

Baines, M., D. J. Oliver, and R. L. Carter. 1985. Medical management of intestinal obstruction in patients with advanced malignant disease: A clinical and pathological study. *Lancet* 2:990–93

Baker, A. R. 1989. Treatment of malignant ascites. In *Cancer: Principles and practice of oncology*, ed. V. T. DeVita, S. Hellman, and S. A. Rosenberg, chapter 62, section 6. Philadelphia: J.B. Lippincott.

Bale, S., and C. Regnard. 1989. Pressure sores in advanced disease: A flow diagram. *Palliative Medicine* 3:263–65.

Barr, H., and N. Krasner. 1991. Prospective quality of life analysis after palliative photoablation for the treatment of malignant dysphagia. *Cancer* 68:1660–64.

Bell, M. D. D., P. Mishra, B. D. Weldon, G. R. Murray, T. N. Calvey, and N. E. Williams. 1985. Buccal morphine: A new route for analgesia? *Lancet* 1:71–73.

Bergner, M., L. D. Hudson, D. A. Conrad, C. M. Patmont, G. J. McDonald, E. B. Perrin, and B. S. Gibson. 1988. The cost and efficacy of home care for patients with chronic lung disease. *Medical Care* 26:566–79.

Berry, J. I. 1988. The use of analgesics in patients with pain from terminal disease. *American Journal of Hospice Care* 5:26–42.

Blum, J. D. 1990. The legal dilemma of stopping artificial feeding. *American Journal of Hospice and Palliative Care* 7:42–48.

Bono, B., P. Cazzaniga, V. Pini, S. M. Zurrida, R. Spagnolo, L. Torelli, C. Corona, and A. Bono. 1991. Palliative surgery of metastatic bone disease: A review of 83 cases. *European Journal of Cancer* 27:556–58.

Brechling, B. G., and D. Kuhn. 1989. A specialized hospice for dementia patients and their families. *American Journal of Hospice Care* 6:27–30.

Breitbart, W. 1987. Suicide in cancer patients. *Oncology* 1:49–54.

Brown, J. H., P. Henteleff, S. Barakat, and C. J. Rowe. 1986. Is it normal for terminally ill patients to desire death? *American Journal of Psychiatry* 143:208–11.

Bruera, E., and N. MacDonald. 1986. Intractable pain in patients with advanced head and neck tumors: a possible role of local infection. *Cancer Treatment Reports* 70:691–92.

Bruera, E., C. Brenneis, M. Michaud, S. Chadwick, and N. MacDonald. 1987. Continuous SC infusion of narcotics using a portable disposable device in patients with advanced cancer. *Cancer Treatment Reports* 71:635–37.

Bruera, E., C. Brenneis, M. Michaud, P. I. Jackson, and R. N. MacDonald. 1988. Muscle electrophysiology in patients with advanced breast cancer. *Journal of the National Cancer Institute* 80:282–85.

Bruera, E., C. Brenneis, M. Michaud, and N. MacDonald. 1987. Continuous SC infusion of metoclopramede for treatment of narcotic bowel syndrome. *Cancer Treatment Reports* 71:1121–22.

Bruera, E., S. Carraro, E. Roca, M. Barugel, and R. Chacon. 1986. Double-blind evaluation of the effects of mazindol on pain, depression, anxiety, appetite, and activity in terminal cancer patients. *Cancer Treatment Reports* 70:295–98.

Bruera, E., S. Chadwick, C. Brenneis, J. Hanson, and N. MacDonald. 1987. Methylphenidate associated with narcotics for the treatment of cancer pain. *Cancer Treatment Reports* 71:67–70.

Bruera, E., S. Chadwick, R. Fox, J. Hanson, and N. MacDonald. 1986. Study of cardiovascular autonomic insufficiency in advanced cancer patients. *Cancer Treatment Reports* 70:1383–87.

Bruera, E., S. Chadwick, A. Weinlick, and N. MacDonald. 1987. Delirium and severe sedation in patients with terminal cancer. *Cancer Treatment Reports* 71:787–88.

Bruera, E., M. A. Legris, N. Kuehn, and M. J. Miller. 1990. Hypodermoclysis for the administration of fluids and narcotic analgesics in patients with advanced cancer. *Journal of Pain and Symptom Management* 5:218–20.

Bruera E., E. Roca, L. Cedaro, S. Carraro, and R. Chacon. 1985. Action of oral methylprednisolone in terminal cancer patients: A prospective randomized double-blind study. *Cancer Treatment Reports* 69:751–54.

Brusis, T., and H. Luckhaupt. 1989. Fetor from ulcerated head and neck tumors: Causation and therapy. *Annals of Otology, Rhinology and Laryngology* 98:615–17.

Bunn, P. A., and E. C. Ridgway. 1989. Paraneoplastic syndromes. In *Cancer: Principles and practice of oncology,* eds. V. T. DeVita, S. Hellman, and S. A. Rosenberg, chapter 55. Philadelphia: J.B. Lippincott.

Caplan, R. A., L. B. Ready, R. V Oden, F. A. Matsen, M. L. Nessly, and G. L. Olsson. 1989. Transdermal fentanyl for postoperative pain management: A double-blind placebo study. *Journal of American Medical Association* 260:1036–39.

Carlson, R. W., L. Devich, and R. R. Frank. 1988. Development of a comprehensive support care team for the hopelessly ill on a university hospital medical service. *Journal of the American Medical Association* 259:378–83.

Carter, R. L., M. R. Pittam, and N. S. B. Tanner. 1982. Pain and dysphagia in patients with squamous carcinomas of the head and neck: The role of perineural spread. *Journal of the Royal Society of Medicine* 75:598–606.

Chapman, C. R, and H. F. Hill. 1989. Prolonged morphine self-administration and addiction liability: Evaluation of two theories in a bone marrow transplantation unit. *Cancer* 63:1636–44.

Citron, M. L., A. Johnston-Early, M. Boyer, S. H. Krasnow, M. Hood, and M. H. Cohen. 1986. Patient-controlled analgesic for severe cancer pain. *Archives of Internal Medicine* 146:734–36.

Clarke, C., I. McConachie, J. D. Edwards, and P. Nightingale. 1990. Concealed haemorrhage in patients nursed on an air-fluidised bed. *British Medical Journal* 301:432.

Cody, M. 1990. Depression and the use of antidepressants in patients with cancer. *Palliative Medicine* 4:271–78.

Colburn, L. 1987. Pressure ulceration prevention for the hospice patient. *American Journal of Hospice Care* 4:22–26.

Cole, R. M. 1991. Medical aspects of care for the person with advanced acquired immunodeficiency syndrome (AIDS): A palliative care perspective. *Palliative Medicine* 5:96–111.

Consensus Conference. 1989. Urinary incontinence in adults. *Journal of the American Medical Association* 261:2685–90.

Cooke, N. 1989. Dyspnea. In *Symptom control*, ed. T. D. Walsh, chapter 14. Boston: Blackwell Scientific Publications.

Council on Ethical and Judicial Affairs. 1991. Guidelines for the appropriate use of do-not-resuscitate orders. *Journal of the American Medical Association* 265:1868–71.

Cousins, M. J., and L. E. Mather. 1984. Intrathecal and epidural administration of opioids. *Anesthesiology* 61:276–310.

Coyle, N., J. Adelhardt, K. M. Foley, and R. K. Portenoy. 1990. Character of terminal illness in the advanced cancer patient: Pain and other symptoms during the last four weeks of life. *Journal of Pain and Symptom Management* 5:83–93.

Coyle, N., A. Mauskop, J. Maggard, and K. M. Foley. 1986. Continuous subcutaneous infusions of opiates in cancer patients with pain. *Oncology Nursing Forum* 13:53–57.

Curtis, E. B., R. Krech, and T. D. Walsh. 1991. Common symptoms in patients with advanced cancer. *Journal of Palliative Care* 7:25–29.

Della Cuna, G. R., A. Pellegrini, and M. Piazzi. 1989. Effect of methylprednisolone sodium succinate on quality of life in preterminal cancer patients: A placebo-controlled, multicenter study. *European Journal of Cancer and Clinical Oncology* 25:1817–21.

Derogatis, L. R., and R. N. MacDonald. 1982. Psychopharmacologic applications to cancer. *Cancer* 50:1968–73.

Derogatis, L. R., G. R. Morrow, J. Fetting, D. Penman, S. Piasetsky, A. M. Schmale, M. Henrichs, and C. L. M. Carnicke. 1983. The prevalence of psychiatric disorders among cancer patients. *Journal of the American Medical Association* 249:751–57.

DeWys, W. D., C. Begg, P. T. Lavin, P. R. Band, J. M. Bennett, J. R. Bertino, M. H. Cohen, H. O. Douglass, P. F. Engstrom, E. Z. Ezdinli, J. Horton, G. J. Johnson, C. G. Moertel, M. M. Oken, C. Perlia, C. Rosenbaum, M. N. Silverstein, R. T. Skeel, R. W. Sponzo, and D. C. Tormey. 1980. Prognostic effect of weight loss prior to chemotherapy in cancer patients. *American Journal of Medicine* 69:491–97.

DeWys, W. D., and F. A. Hoffman. 1984. Pathophysiology of anorexia and disturbances of taste in cancer patients. In *Frontiers in gastrointestinal cancer*, eds. B. Levin and R. H. Riddell, 81–90. New York: Elsevier.

Dodds, L. J. 1985. The control of cancer chemotherapy-induced nausea and vomiting. *Journal of Clinical and Hospital Pharmacy* 10:143–66.

Duffield, M. 1989. Bedsores. In: *Symptom control*, ed. T. D. Walsh, chapter 4. Boston: Blackwell Scientific Publications.

Duffy, T. P. 1992. Clinical problem-solving. *New England Journal of Medicine* 326:933–35.

DuPen, S. L., D. G. Peterson, A. C. Bogosian, D. H. Ramsey, C. Larson, and M.

Omoto. 1987. A new permanent exteriorized epidural catheter for narcotic self-administration to control cancer pain. *Cancer* 59:986–93.

Duthie, D. J. R., and W. S. Nimmo. 1987. Adverse effects of opioid analgesic drugs. *British Journal of Anaesthesiology* 59:61–77.

Editorial. 1986. Spinal opiates revisited. *Lancet* 1:655–56.

Editorial. 1986. Terminal dehydration. *Lancet* 1:306.

Editorial. 1990. Management of smelly tumours. *Lancet* 335:141–42.

Editorial. 1990. Strontium and bone pain. *Lancet* 335:384–85.

Editorial. 1992. Endoprosthesis for bone metastases. *Lancet* 339:1145.

Ellison, N. M., and G. O. Lewis. 1984. Plasma concentrations following single doses of morphine sulfate in oral solution and rectal suppository. *Clinical Pharmacy* 3:614–17.

Enck, R. E. 1991. Pain control in the ambulatory elderly. *Geriatrics* 46:49–60.

Enck, R. E. 1992. A review of pain management. *American Journal of Hospice and Palliative Care* 9:6–12.

Enck, R. E., D. R. Longa, M. W. Arren, and B. A. McCann. 1988. DNR Policies in healthcare organizations with emphasis on hospice. *American Journal of Hospice Care* 5:39–42.

Estenne, M., J. C. Yernault, and A. DeTroyer. 1983. Mechanism of relief of dyspnea after thoracocentesis in patients with large pleural effusions. *American Journal of Medicine* 74:813–19.

Evans, A. L., and B. A. Brody. 1985. The do-not-resuscitate order in teaching hospitals. *Journal of the American Medical Association* 253:2236–39.

Evans, C., and M. McCarthy. 1985. Prognostic uncertainty in terminal care: Can the Karnofsky index help? *Lancet* 1:1204–6.

Faber-Langendoen, K. 1991. Resuscitation of patients with metastatic cancer: Is transient benefit still futile? *Archives of Internal Medicine* 151:235–39.

Fainsinger, R., M. J. Miller, E. Bruera, J. Hanson, and T. MacEachern. 1991. Symptom control during the last week of life on a palliative care unit. *Journal of Palliative Care* 7:5–11.

Fainsinger, R. L., and E. Bruera. 1991. Hypodermoclysis (HDC) for symptom control vs. the Edmonton injector (EI). *Journal of Palliative Care* 7:5–8.

Fabiszewski, K. J., B. Volicer, and L. Volicer. 1990. Effect of antibiotic treatment on outcome of fevers in institutionalized Alzheimer patients. *Journal of the American Medical Association* 263:3168–72.

Ferrer-Brechner, T. 1989. Anesthetic techniques for the management of cancer pain. *Cancer* 63:2343–47.

Ferris, F. D. 1990. Pre-terminal delirium. In *A Practical Seminar/Workshop on Narcotic Infusions*, ed. F. D. Ferris, 25–28. Toronto: Pain Management Group.

Filshie, J., and P. J. Morrison. 1988. Acupuncture for chronic pain: A review. *Palliative Medicine* 2:1–14.

Filshie, J., and D. Redman. 1985. Acupuncture and malignant pain problems. *European Journal of Surgical Oncology* 11:389–94.

Finlay, I. G. 1986. Oral symptoms and candida in the terminally ill. *British Medical Journal* 292:592–93.

Foley, K. M. 1985. The treatment of cancer pain. *New England Journal of Medicine* 313:84–95.

Foley, K. M. 1989. Controversies in cancer pain: Medical perspectives. *Cancer* 63:2257–65.

Foley, K. M., and E. Arbit. 1989. Management of cancer pain. In *Cancer: Principles and practice of oncology*, eds. V. T. DeVita, S. Hellman, and S. A. Rosenberg, chapter 59, section 4. Philadelphia: J.B. Lippincott.

Foley, K. M., and C. E. Inturrisi. 1987. Analgesic drug therapy in cancer pain: Principles and practice. *Medical Clinics of North America* 71:207–32.

Forbes, J. F. 1988. Principles and potential of palliative surgery in patients with advanced cancer. In *Supportive care in cancer patients*, eds. H. J. Senn, A. Glaus, and L. Schmid, 134–42. New York: Springer-Verlag.

Forrest, W. H., B. W. Brown, C. R. Brown, R. Defalque, M. Gold, H. E. Gordon, K. E. James, J. Katz, D. L. Mahler, P. Schroff, and G. Teutsch. 1977. Dextroamphetamine with morphine for the treatment of postoperative pain. *New England Journal of Medicine* 296:712–15.

Forster, L. E., and J. Lynn. 1988. Predicting life span for applicants to inpatient hospice. *Archives of Internal Medicine* 148:2540–43.

Forster, L. E., and J. Lynn. 1989. The use of physiologic measures and demographic variables to predict longevity among inpatient hospice applicants. *American Journal of Hospice Care* 6:31–34.

Frytak, S., and C. G. Moertel. 1981. Management of nausea and vomiting in the cancer patient. *Journal of the American Medical Association* 245:393–96.

Glass, R. M. 1983. Psychiatric disorders among cancer patients. *Journal of the American Medical Association* 249:782–83.

Gold, J. W. M. 1992. HIV-1 infection. Diagnosis and management. *Medical Clinics of North America* 76:1–18.

Greco, P. J., K. A. Schulman, R. Lavizzo-Mourey, and J. Hansen-Flaschen. 1991. The patient self-determination act and the future of advance directives. *Annals of Internal Medicine* 115:639–43.

Greene, W. R., and W. H. Davis. 1991. Titrated intravenous barbiturates in the control of symptoms in patients with terminal cancer. *Southern Medical Journal* 84:332–37.

Gregory, R. E., S. A. Grossman, V. R. Sheidler, and L. E. Wiggins. 1991. Seizures (SZ) associated with high-dose, intravenous (IV) morphine (MS) infusions: Incidence and possible etiology. *Proceedings of American Society of Clinical Oncology* 10:335 (abstract).

Hanks, G. W. 1984. Psychotropic drugs. *Clinics in Oncology* 3:135–51.

Hanks, G. W. 1989. Controlled-release morphine (MST Contin) in advanced cancer: The European experience. *Cancer* 63:2378–82.

Hanks, G. W., and D. M. Justins. 1992. Cancer pain: Management. *Lancet* 339:1031–36.

Hanson, D., D. K. Langemo, B. Olson, S. Hunter, T. R. Sauvage, C. Burd, and T. Cathcart-Silberberg. 1991. The prevalence and incidence of pressure ulcers in the hospice setting: Analysis of two methodologies. *American Journal of Hospice and Palliative Care* 8:18–22.

Heilmann, K. 1978. Therapeutic systems for systemic use. In *Therapeutic systems. Pattern-specific drug delivery: Concept and development*, ed. K. Heilmann, 43–77. Stuttgart: Georg Thieme.

Henry, K., S. Rathgaber, C. Sullivan, and K. McCabe. 1992. Diabetes mellitus induced by megestrol acetate in a patient with AIDS and cachexia. *Annals of Internal Medicine* 116:53–54.

Herwig, K. R. 1980. Management of urinary incontinence and retention in the patient with advanced cancer. *Journal of the American Medical Association* 244:2203–4.

Higginson, I., and M. McCarthy. 1989. Measuring symptoms in terminal cancer: Are pain and dyspnea controlled? *Journal of the Royal Society of Medicine* 82:264–67.

Higginson, I., A. Wade, and M. McCarthy. 1990. Financial help for terminally ill patients. *Lancet* 1:172.

Hockley, J. M., R. Dunlop, and R. J. Davies. 1988. Survey of distressing symptoms in dying patients and their families in hospital and the response to a symptom control team. *British Medical Journal* 296:1715–17.

Hoffman, M., A. Provatas, A. Lyver, and R. Kanner. 1991. Pain management in the opioid-addicted patient with cancer. *Cancer* 68:1121–22.

Hogan, C. M. 1986. Nausea and vomiting. In *Nursing Management of Symptoms Associated with Chemotherapy*, ed. J. M. Yasko, 57–71. Columbus, Ohio: Adria Laboratories.

Hogan, Q., D. E. Weissman, J. D. Haddox, S. Abram, M. L. Taylor, and N. Janjan. 1991. Epidural opiates and local anesthetics for the management of cancer pain. *Proceedings of the American Society of Clinical Oncology* 10:329 (abstract).

Holland, J. C. 1987. Managing depression in the patient with cancer. *CA: A Cancer Journal for Clinicians* 37:366–71.

Holland, J. C., G. R. Morrow, A. Schmale, L. Derogatis, M. Stefanek, S. Berenson, P. J. Carpenter, W. Breitbart, and M. Feldstein. 1991. A randomized clinical trial of alprazolam versus progressive muscle relaxation in cancer patients with anxiety and depressive symptoms. *Journal of Clinical Oncology* 9:1004–11.

Holmes, V. F., F. Adams, and F. Fernandez. 1987. Respiratory dyskinesia due to antiemetic therapy in a cancer patient. *Cancer Treatment Reports* 71:415–16.

Hoskin, P. J., and G. W. Hanks. 1988. The management of symptoms in advanced cancer: Experience in a hospital-based continuing care unit. *Journal of the Royal Society of Medicine* 81:341–44.

Hoskin, P. J., and G. W. Hanks. 1990. Morphine: Pharmacokinetics and clinical practice. *British Journal of Cancer* 62:705–7.

Humphry, D. 1991. *Final exit*. Eugene, Oreg.: The Hemlock Society.

Jacobsberg, L. B., and S. Perry. 1992. Psychiatric disturbances. *Medical Clinics of North America* 76:99–106.

Jaffe, J. H. 1985. Drug addiction and drug abuse. In *The pharmacological basis of therapeutics*, eds. A. G. Gilman, L. S. Goodman, T. W. Rall, and F. Murad, chapter 23. New York: Macmillan.

Johanson, G. A. 1992. New routes of opioid administration. *American Journal of Hospice and Palliative Care* 9:4–5.

Joshi, J. H., C. A. deJongh, N. Schnaper, C. L. Fortner, and P. H. Wiernik. 1982. Amphetamine therapy for enhancing the comfort of terminally ill patients (pts) with cancer. *Proceedings of the American Society of Clinical Oncology* 1:55 (abstract).

Kaiko, R. F., S. L. Wallenstein, A. G. Rogers, P. Y. Grabinski, and R. W. Houde. 1982. Narcotics in the elderly. *Medical Clinics of North America* 66:1079–89.

Kaplan, L. D., C. B. Wofsy, and P. A. Volberding. 1987. Treatment of patients with acquired immunodeficiency syndrome and associated manifestations. *Journal of the American Medical Association* 257:1367–74.

Karnofsky, D. A., and J. H. Burchenal. 1949. The clinical evaluation of chemotherapeutic agents in cancer. In *Evaluation of chemotherapeutic agents*, ed. C. M. Macleod, 191–205. New York: Columbia University Press.

Kellar, M. 1984. A retrospective review of patients receiving continuous morphine infusion. *PRN Forum* 3:5–6.

Kerr, D. 1989. A bedside fan for terminal dyspnea. *American Journal of Hospice Care* 6:22.

Kerr, I. G., M. Sone, C. DeAngelis, N. Iscoe, R. MacKenzie, and T. Schueller. 1988. Continuous narcotic infusion with patient-controlled analgesia for chronic cancer pain in outpatients. *Annals of Internal Medicine* 108:554–57.

Kevorkian, J. 1991. *Prescription: Medicide.* Buffalo: Prometheus Books.

Kinzel, T. 1991. Managing lung disease in late life: A new approach. *Geriatrics* 46:54–59.

Krebs, H. B., and D. R. Goplerud. 1983. Surgical management of bowel obstruction in advanced ovarian carcinoma. *Obstetrics and Gynecology* 61:327–30.

Kris, M. G., S. D. J. Yeh, R. J. Gralla, and C. W. Young. 1985. Symptomatic gastroparesis in cancer patients: A possible cause of cancer-associated anorexia that can be improved with oral metoclopramide. *Proceedings of the American Society of Clinical Oncology* 4:267 (abstract).

Lamerton, R. 1991. Dehydration in dying patients. *Lancet* 337:981–82.

Langstein, H. N., and J. A. Norton. 1991. Mechanisms of cancer cachexia. *Hematology/Oncology Clinics of North America* 5:103–23.

Levick, S., C. Jacobs, D. F. Loukas, D. H. Gordon, F. L. Meyskens, and K. Uhm. 1988. Naproxen sodium in treatment of bone pain due to metastatic cancer. *Pain* 35:253–58.

Levine, P. M., P. M. Silberfarb, and Z. J. Lipowski. 1978. Mental disorders in cancer patients: A study of 100 psychiatric referrals. *Cancer* 42:1385–91.

Levy, D. E., J. J. Caronna, B. H. Singer, R. H. Lapinski, H. Frydman, and F.Plum. 1985. Predicting outcome from hypoxic-ischemic coma. *Journal of the American Medical Association* 253:1420–26.

Librach, S. L., and L. M. Rapson. 1988. The use of transcutaneous electrical nerve stimulation (TENS) for the relief of pain in palliative care. *Palliative Medicine* 2:15–20.

Lichter, I. 1990. Weakness in terminal illness. *Palliative Medicine* 4:73–80.

Lichter, I., and E. Hunt. 1990. The last 48 hours of life. *Journal of Palliative Care* 6:7–15.

Lindley, C. M., J. A. Dalton, and S. M. Fields. 1990. Narcotic analgesics: Clinical pharmacology and therapeutics. *Cancer Nursing* 13:28–38.

Lipman, A. G. 1989. Opioid analgesics in the management of cancer pain. *American Journal of Hospice Care* 6:13–23.

Lipowski, Z. J. 1987. Delirium (acute confusional states). *Journal of the American Medical Association* 258:1789–92.

Lipowski, Z. J. 1989. Delirium in the elderly patient. *New England Journal of Medicine* 320:578–82.

Lo, B. 1991. Unanswered questions about DNR orders. *Journal of the American Medical Association* 265:1874–75.

Longstreth, W. T., T. S. Inui, L. A. Cobb, and M. K. Copass. 1983. Neurologic recovery after out-of-hospital cardiac arrest. *Annals of Internal Medicine* 98:588–92.

Loprinzi, C. L., N. M., Ellison, D. J. Schaid, J. E. Krook, L. M. Athmann, A. M. Dose, J. A. Mailliard, P. S. Johnson, L. P. Ebbert, and L. H. Geeraerts. 1990. Controlled trial of megestrol acetate for the treatment of cancer anorexia and cachexia. *Journal of National Cancer Institute* 82:1127–32.

Loprinzi, C. L., J. Mailliard, D. J. Schaid, J. E. Krook, R. M. Goldberg, M. Keppen, and J. Michalak. 1992. Dose/response evaluation of megestrol acetate (MA) for the treatment of cancer anorexia/cachexia: A Mayo Clinic and North Central Cancer Treatment Group Trial. *Proceedings of the American Society of Clinical Oncology* 11:378 (abstract).

Lynn, J. 1986. Dying and dementia. *Journal of the American Medical Association* 256:2244–45.

McNamara, P., M. Minton, and R. G. Twycross. 1991. Use of midazolam in palliative care. *Palliative Medicine* 5:244–49.

Magni, G., P. Conlon, and D. Arsie. 1987. Tricyclic antidepressants in the treatment of cancer pain: A review. *Pharmacopsychiatry* 20:160–64.

Maguire, L. C., J. L. Yon, and E. Miller. 1981. Prevention of narcotic induced constipation. *New England Journal of Medicine* 305:1651 (letter).

Maloney, C. M., R. K. Kesner, G. Klein, and J. Bockenstette. 1989. The rectal administration of MS Contin: Clinical implications of use in end stage cancer. *American Journal of Hospice Care* 6:34–35.

Maouskop, A., N. Coyle, J. Maggard, and K. M. Foley. 1985. Continuous subcutaneous infusions of opiates in cancer patients with pain: Safety and efficacy. *Proceedings of the American Society of Clinical Oncology* 4:39 (abstract).

Marin, J., M. C. Ilanez, and S. Arribas. 1990. Therapeutic management of nausea and vomiting. *General Pharmacology* 21:1–10.

Massie, M. J., J. Holland, and E. Glass. 1983. Delirium in terminally ill cancer patients. *American Journal of Psychiatry* 140:1048–50.

Medical Letter. 1989a. Drugs that cause psychiatric symptoms. *Medical Letter* 31:113–18.

Medical Letter. 1989b. Drugs for rheumatoid arthritis. *Medical Letter* 31:61–64.

Melzack, R., B. M. Mount, and J. M. Gordon. 1979. The Brompton mixture versus morphine solution given orally: Effects on pain. *Canadian Medical Association Journal* 120:435–38.

Miser, A. W., P. K. Narang, J. A. Dothage, R. C. Young, W. Sindelar, and J. S. Miser. 1989. Transdermal fentanyl for pain control in patients with cancer. *Pain* 37:15–21.

Mitsumoto, H., M. R. Hanson, and D. A. Chad. 1988. Amyotrophic lateral sclerosis: Recent advances in pathogenesis and therapeutic trials. *Archives of Neurology* 45:189–202.

Moertel, C. G., A. J. Schutt, R. J. Reitemeier, and R. J. Hahn. 1974. Corticosteroid therapy of preterminal gastrointestinal cancer. *Cancer* 33:1607–9.

Morris, J. N., S. Suissa, S. Sherwood, S. M. Wright, and D. Greer. 1986. Last days: A study of the quality of life of terminally ill cancer patients. *Journal of Chronic Disease* 39:47–62.

Moss, V. 1991. Patient characteristics, presentation, and problems encountered in advanced AIDS in a hospice setting: A review. *Palliative Medicine* 5:112–16.

Moulin, D. E., J. H. Kreeft, N. Murray-Parsons, and A. I. Bouquillon. 1991. Comparison of continuous subcutaneous and intravenous hydromorphone infusions for management of cancer pain. *Lancet* 337:465–68.

Newman, V., M. Allwood, and R. A. Oakes. 1989. The use of metronidazole gel to control the smell of malodorous lesions. *Palliative Medicine* 3:303–5.

Nielsen, O. S., A. J. Munro, and I. F. Tannock. 1991. Bone metastases: Pathophysiology and management policy. *Journal of Clinical Oncology* 9:509–24.

O'Brien, T., M. Kelly, and C. Saunders. 1992. Motor neurone disease: A hospice perspective. *British Medical Journal* 304:471–73.

Osteen, R. T., S. Guyton, G. Steele, and R. E. Wilson. 1980. Malignant intestinal obstruction. *Surgery* 87:611–15.

Pass, H. I., and J. A. Roth. 1987. Diagnosis of pulmonary metastases. In *Surgical treatment of metastatic disease*, ed. S. A. Rosenberg, chapter 2. Philadelphia: J.B. Lippincott.

Payne, R. 1987a. Novel routes of opioid administration in the management of cancer pain. *Oncology* 1:10–18.

Payne, R. 1987b. Role of epidural and intrathecal narcotics and peptides in the management of cancer pain. *Medical Clinics of North America* 71:313–27.

Payne, R. 1989a. Novel routes of opioid administration: Part 5. Spinal epidural and intrathecal. *Primary Care and Cancer* 9:31–32.

Payne, R. 1989b. Pharmacologic management of bone pain in the cancer patient. *Clinical Journal of Pain* 5(Suppl. 2):S43–50.

Payne, R. 1991. Pain. In *Manual of oncologic therapeutics, 1991/1992*, ed. R. E. Wittes, chapter 57. Philadelphia: J.B. Lippincott.

Payne, R. 1992. Transdermal fentanyl: Suggested recommendations for clinical use. *Journal of Pain and Symptom Management* 7:s40–s44.

Penn, R. D., and J. A. Paice. 1987. Chronic intrathecal morphine for intractable pain. *Journal of Neurosurgery* 67:182–86.

Peteet, J., V. Tay, G. Cohen, and J. MacIntyre. 1986. Pain characteristics and treatment in an outpatient cancer population. *Cancer* 57:1259–65.

Phillips, H. 1984. Orthopaedic surgery. *Clinics in Oncology* 3:75–87.

Pitorak, E. F., and J. C. Kraus. 1987. Pain control with sublingual morphine: The advantages for hospice care. *American Journal of Hospice Care* 4:39–41.

Plezia, P. M., T. H. Kramer, J. Linford, and S. R. Hameroff. 1989. Transdermal fentanyl: Pharmacokinetics and preliminary clinical evaluation. *Pharmacotherapy* 9:2–9.

Popiela, T., R. Lucchi, and F. Giongo. 1989. Methylprednisolone as palliative therapy for female terminal cancer patients. *European Journal of Cancer and Clinical Oncology* 25:1823–29.

Portenoy, R. K. 1987. Constipation in the cancer patient: Causes and management. *Medical Clinics of North America* 71:303–11.

Portenoy, R. K. 1990. Drug therapy for cancer pain. *American Journal of Hospice and Pallative Care* 7:10–19.

Portenoy, R. K., D. E. Moulin, A. Rogers, C. E. Inturrisi, and K. M. Foley. 1986. IV infusion of opioids for cancer pain: Clinical review and guidelines for use. *Cancer Treatment Reports* 70:575–81.

Posner, J. B. 1979. Neurological complications of systemic cancer. *Medical Clinics of North America* 63:783–800.

Potter, W. Z., M. V. Rudorfer, and H. Manji. 1991. The pharmacologic treatment of depression. *New England Journal of Medicine* 325:633–42.

Poulsen, H. S., O. S. Nielsen, M. Klee, and M. Rorth. 1989. Palliative irradiation of bone metastases. *Cancer Treatment Reviews* 16:41–48.

Powell, N. 1988. Tao: The Chinese way. In *The book of change: How to understand and use the I. Ching*, chapter 1. London: Macdonald and Company.

President's Commission on the Study of Ethical Problems in Medicine and Biomedical and Behavioral Research. 1983. *Deciding to forego life-sustaining treatment: A report on the ethical, medical, and legal issues in the treatment decisions.* Washington, D.C.: U.S. Government Printing Office.

Ray, W. A., M. R. Griffin, W. Schaffner, D. K. Baugh, and L. J. Melton. 1987. Psychotropic drug use and the risk of hip fracture. *New England Journal of Medicine* 316:363–69.

Redfield, R. R., and E. C. Tramont. 1989. Toward a better classification system for HIV infection. *New England Journal of Medicine* 320:1414–16.

Rees, W. D., S. B. Dover, and T. S. Low-Beer. 1987. "Patients with terminal cancer" who have neither terminal illness nor cancer. *British Medical Journal* 295:318–19.

Regnard, C. 1988. The treatment of bowel obstruction in advanced cancer: An algorithm. *Palliative Medicine* 2:131–33.

Regnard, C., and S. Ahmedzai. 1991. Dyspnoea in advanced nonmalignant disease: A flow diagram. *Palliative Medicine* 5:56–60.

Regnard, C., and K. Mannix. 1991. Urinary problems in advanced cancer: A flow diagram. *Palliative Medicine* 5:344–48.

Reitmeier, M., and R. C. Hartenstein. 1990. Megestrolacetate and determination of body composition by bioelectrical impedance analysis in cancer cachexia. *Proceedings of the American Society of Clinical Oncology* 9:325 (abstract).

Reuben, D. B., and V. Mor. 1986a. Dyspnea in terminally ill cancer patients. *Chest* 89:234–36.

Reuben, D. B., and V. Mor. 1986b. Nausea and vomiting in terminal cancer patients. *Archives of Internal Medicine* 146:2021–23.

Reuben, D. B., V. Mor, and J. Hiris. 1988. Clinical symptoms and length of survival in patients with terminal cancer. *Archives of Internal Medicine* 148:1586–91.

Reuler, J. B., and T. G. Cooney. 1981. The pressure sore: Pathophysiology and principles of management. *Annals of Internal Medicine* 94:661–66.

Rivlin, R. S., M. E. Shils, and P. Sherlock. 1983. Nutrition and cancer. *American Journal of Medicine* 75:843–54.

Rowland, C. G., and K. M. Pagliero. 1985. Intracavitary irradiation in palliation of carcinoma of oesophagus and cardia. *Lancet* 2:981–83.

Rowlingson, J. C., R. J. Hamill, and R. B. Patt. 1993. Comprehensive assessment of the patient with cancer pain. In *Cancer pain*, ed. R. B. Patt, chapter 2. Philadelphia: J.B. Lippincott.

Roy, D. J. 1991. Need they sleep before they die? *Journal of Palliative Care* 6:3–4.

Ryan, T. J. 1989. Pressure sores: Prevention, management and future research—a medical perspective. *Palliative Medicine* 3:249–55.

Sandgren, J. E., M. S. McPhee, and N. J. Greenberger. 1984. Narcotic bowel syndrome treated with clonidine: Resolution of abdominal pain and intestinal pseudo-obstruction. *Annals of Internal Medicine* 101:331–34.

Saunders, C. 1982. Principles of symptom control in terminal care. *Medical Clinics of North America* 66:1169–83.

Saunders, C. 1989. Pain and impending death. In *Textbook of pain*, eds. P. D. Wall and R. Melzack, 624–31. Edinburgh: Churchill Livingstone.

Saunders, C., T. D. Walsh, and M. Smith. 1981. Hospice care in motor neuron disease. In *Hospice: The living idea*, eds. C. Saunders, D. H. Summers, and N. Teller, chapter 6. London: Edward Arnold.

Sawe, J., B. Dahlstrom, L. Paalzow, and A. Rane. 1981. Morphine kinetics in cancer patients. *Clinical Pharmacology and Therapeutics* 30:629–35.

Schell, H. W. 1972. Adrenal corticosteroid therapy in far-advanced cancer. *Geriatrics* 27:131–41.

Seigel, L. J., and D. L. Longo. 1981. The control of chemotherapy-induced emesis. *Annals of Internal Medicine* 95:352–59.

Sharp, K. W., and E. J. Stevens. 1991. Improving palliation in pancreatic cancer: Intraoperative celiac plexus block for pain relief. *Southern Medical Journal* 84:469–71.

Silverstein, M. D., C. B. Stocking, J. P. Antel, J. Beckwith, R. P. Roos, and M. Seigler. 1991. Amyotrophic lateral sclerosis and life-sustaining therapy: Patients' desires for information, participation in decision making and life-sustaining therapy. *Mayo Clinic Proceedings* 66:906–13.

Simmonds, M. A., R. Payne, J. Richenbacher, K. Moran, and M. A. Southam.

1989. TTS (fentanyl) in the management of pain in patients with cancer. *Proceedings of the American Society of Clinical Oncology* 8:324 (abstract).

Socher, S. H., D. Martinez, J. B. Craig, J. G. Kuhn, and A. Oliff. 1988. Tumor necrosis factor not detectable in patients with clinical cancer cachexia. *Journal of National Cancer Institute* 80:595–98.

Sorensen, P. S., S. E. Borgesen, K. Rohde, B. Rasmusson, F. Bach, T. Boge-Rasmussen, P. Stjernholm, B. H. Larson, N. Agerlin, and F. Gjerris. 1990. Metastatic epidural spinal cord compression: Results of treatment and survival. *Cancer* 65:1502–8.

Stedeford, A., and C. Regnard. 1991. Confusional states in advanced cancer: A flow diagram. *Palliative Medicine* 5:256–61.

Steiner, I., and T. Siegal. 1989. Muscle cramps in cancer patients. *Cancer* 63:574–77.

Steitz, A. M. 1987. Analgesic utilization patterns in a hospice. *Oncology* 1:33–36.

Sugibayashi, K., C. Sakanoue, and Y. Morimoto. 1989. Utility of topical formulations of morphine hydrochloride containing azone and N-methyl-2-pyrrolidone. *Selective Cancer Therapeutics* 5:119–28.

Sundaresan, N., G. V. DiGiacinto, and J. E. O. Hughes. 1989. Neurosurgery in the treatment of cancer pain. *Cancer* 63:2365–77.

Swanson, G., J. Smith, R. Bulich, P. New, and R. Shiffman. 1989. Patient-controlled analgesia for chronic cancer pain in the ambulatory setting: A report of 117 patients. *Journal of Clinical Oncology* 7:1903–8.

Sykes, N. P. 1991. A clinical comparison of laxatives in a hospice. *Palliative Medicine* 5:307–14.

Sykes, N. P., R. L. Carter, and M. Baines. 1988. Clinical and pathological study of dysphagia conservatively managed in patients with advanced malignant disease. *Lancet* 2:726–28.

Tannock, I., M. Gospodarowicz, W. Meakin, T. Panzarella, L. Stewart, and W. Rider. 1989. Treatment of metastatic prostatic cancer with low-dose prednisone: Evaluation of pain and quality of life as pragmatic indices of response. *Journal of Clinical Oncology* 7:590–97.

Tchekmedyian, N. S., N. Tait, M. Moody, and J. Aisner. 1987. High-dose megestrol acetate: A possible treatment for cachexia. *Journal of the American Medical Association* 257:1195–98.

Temple, W. J., and A. S. Ketcham. 1990. Surgical palliation for recurrent rectal cancers ulcerating in the perineum. *Cancer* 65:1111–14.

Thirlwell, M. P., P. A. Sloan, J. A. Maroun, G. J. Boors, J. G. Besner, J. H. Stewart, and B. M. Mount. 1989. Pharmacokinetics and clinical efficacy of oral morphine solution and controlled-release morphine tablets in cancer patients. *Cancer* 63:2275–83.

Toscani, F., K. Barosi, S. Camerini, and M. Gallucci. 1989. Sodium naproxen: Continuous subcutaneous infusion in neoplastic pain control. *Palliative Medicine* 3:207–11.

Turnbull, A. D. M., J. Guerra, and H. F. Starnes. 1989. Results of surgery for obstructing carcinomatosis of gastrointestinal, pancreatic or biliary origin. *Journal of Clinical Oncology* 7:381–86.

Twycross, R. G., and G. W. Hanks. 1984. Co-analgesia. *Clinics in Oncology* 3:153–64.

U.S. General Accounting Office. 1989. Hospice participation in Medicare: Executive summary. In *GAO/HRD-89–111 Hospice participation in Medicare*, 2–5. Washington D.C.: U.S. Government Printing Office.

Van Holten-Verzantvoort, A. T., O. L. M. Bijvoet, J. Hermans, H. I. J.Harinck, J. W. F. Elte, L. V. A. M. Beex, F. J. Cleton, H. M. Kroon, P. Vermey, J. P. Neijt, and G. Blijham. 1987. Reduced morbidity from skeletal metastases in breast cancer patients during long-term biphosphonate (APD) treatment. *Lancet* 2:983–85.

Veith, I. 1972. *The yellow emperor's classic of internal medicine.* Berkeley and Los Angeles: University of California Press.

Ventafridda, V., C. Ripamonti, A. Caraceni, E. Spoldi, L. Messina, and F. DeConno. 1990. The management of inoperable gastrointestinal obstruction in terminal cancer patients. *Tumori* 76:389–93.

Ventafridda, V., C. Ripamonti, F. DeConno, M. Tamburini, and B. R. Cassileth. 1990. Symptom prevalence and control during cancer patients' last days of life. *Journal of Palliative Care* 6:7–11.

Ventafridda, V., M. Tamburini, A. Caraceni, F. DeConno, and F. Naldi. 1987. A validation study of the WHO method for cancer pain relief. *Cancer* 59:850–56.

Veronesi, V. 1982. Noncurative surgery. In *Cancer Medicine*, eds. J. F. Holland and E. Frei, section IX-4. Philadelphia: Lea and Febiger.

Volicer, L., Y. Rheaume, J. Brown, K. Fabiszewski, and R. Brady. 1986. Hospice approach to the treatment of patients with advanced dementia of the Alzheimer type. *Journal of the American Medical Association* 256:2210–13.

Von Roenn, J. H., R. L. Murphy, K. M. Weber, L. M. Williams, and S. A. Weitzman. 1988. Megestrol acetate for treatment of cachexia associated with human immunodeficiency virus (HIV) infection. *Annals of Internal Medicine* 109:840–41.

Von Roenn, J. H., R. L. Murphy, and N. Wegener. 1990. Megestrol acetate for treatment of anorexia and cachexia associated with human immunodeficiency virus infection. *Seminars in Oncology* 6(Suppl. 9):13–16.

Wadleigh, R., M. Spaulding, B. Lembersky, M. Zimmer, K. Shepard, and T. Plasse. 1990. Dronabinol enhancement of appetite in cancer patients. *Proceedings of the American Society of Clinical Oncology* 9:331 (abstract).

Waller, A., A. Adunski, and M. Hershkowitz. 1991. Terminal dehydration and intravenous fluids. *Lancet* 337:745.

Walsh, J. S., G. Welch, and E. B. Larson. 1990. Survival of outpatients with Alzheimer-type dementia. *Annals of Internal Medicine* 113:429–34.

Warrington, P. S., S. G. Allan, M. A. Cornbleet, J. S. MacPherson, J. F. Smyth, and R. C. F. Leonard. 1986. Optimizing antiemesis in cancer chemotherapy: Efficacy of continuous versus intermittent infusion of high dose metoclopramide in emesis induced by cisplatin. *British Medical Journal* 293:1334–37.

Watson, C. P., R. J. Evans, K. Reed, H. Merskey, L. Goldsmith, and J. Warsh.

1982. Amitriptyline versus placebo in postherpetic neuralgia. *Neurology* 32:671–73.

Weiss, S. H. 1992. HIV infection and the healthcare worker. *Medical Clinics of North America* 76:269–280.

Weissman, D. E., J. L. Dahl, and D. E. Joranson. 1990. Oral morphine for the treatment of cancer pain. *Principles and Practice of Oncology Updates* 6:1–8.

Weissman, D. E, D. E. Joranson, and M. Hopwood. 1991. The influence of drug regulations on opioid analgesic prescribing practice. *Proceedings of the American Society of Clinical Oncology* 10:321 (abstract).

Wells, J. C. D. 1989. The use of nerve destruction for relief of pain in cancer: A review. *Palliative Medicine* 3:239–47.

White, I. D., P. J. Hoskins, G. W. Hanks, and J. M. Bliss. 1989. Morphine and dryness of the mouth. *British Medical Journal* 298:1222–23.

White, I. D., P. J. Hoskins, G. W. Hanks, and J. M. Bliss. 1991. Analysis in cancer pain: Current practice and beliefs. *British Journal of Cancer* 63:271–74.

White, P. F. 1988. Use of patient-controlled analgesia for management of acute pain. *Journal of the American Medical Association* 259:243–47.

Wilkes, E. 1974. Some problems in cancer management. *Proceedings of the Royal Society of Medicine* 67:1001–5.

Williams, D. B., and A. J. Windebank. 1991. Motor neuron disease (amyotrophic lateral sclerosis). *Mayo Clinic Proceedings* 66:54–82.

Willox, J. C., J. Corr, J. Shaw, M. Richardson, K. C. Calman, and M. Drennan. 1984. Prednisolone as an appetite stimulant in patients with cancer. *British Medical Journal* 288:27.

Wolf, S. M., P. Boyle, D. Callahan, J. J. Fins, B. Jennings, J. L. Nelson, J. A. Barondess, D. W. Brock, R. Dresser, L. Emanuel, S. Johnson, J. Lantos, D. R. Mason, M. Mezey, D. Orentlicher, and F. Rouse. 1991. Sources of concern about the Patient Self-Determination Act. *New England Journal of Medicine* 325:1666–71.

Wood, D. K. 1980. The draining malignant ulceration: Palliative management in advanced cancer. *Journal of the American Medical Association* 244:820–22.

Wrenn, K. 1989. Fecal impaction. *New England Journal of Medicine* 321:658–62.

Yarchoan, R., and S. Broder. 1987. Development of antiretroviral therapy for the acquired immunodeficiency syndrome and related disorders. *New England Journal of Medicine* 316:557–64.

Yates, J. W., B. Chalmer, and F. P. McKegney. 1980. Evaluation of patients with advanced cancer using the Karnofsky performance status. *Cancer* 45:2220–24.

Zerwekh, J. V. 1987. Should fluid and nutritional support be withheld from terminally ill patients? Another opinion. *American Journal of Hospice Care* 4:37–38.

Index